# Lecture Notes in Computer Science 14315

## Founding Editors

Gerhard Goos

Juris Hartmanis

## Editorial Board Members

The series Lecture Notes in Computer Science (LNCS), including its subseries Lecture Notes in Artificial Intelligence (LNAI) and Lecture Notes in Bioinformatics (LNBI), has established itself as a medium for the publication of new developments in computer science and information technology research, teaching, and education.

LNCS enjoys close cooperation with the computer science R & D community, the series counts many renowned academics among its volume editors and paper authors, and collaborates with prestigious societies. Its mission is to serve this international community by providing an invaluable service, mainly focused on the publication of conference and workshop proceedings and postproceedings. LNCS commenced publication in 1973.

Andreas K. Maier · Julia A. Schnabel ·
Pallavi Tiwari · Oliver Stegle
Editors

# Machine Learning for Multimodal Healthcare Data

First International Workshop, ML4MHD 2023
Honolulu, Hawaii, USA, July 29, 2023
Proceedings

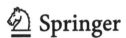 Springer

*Editors*
Andreas K. Maier 🆔
Friedrich-Alexander-Universität
Erlangen-Nürnberg
Erlangen, Bayern, Germany

Pallavi Tiwari 🆔
College of Engineering
University of Wisconsin–Madison
Madison, WI, USA

Julia A. Schnabel 🆔
Technical University of Munich
Garching bei München, Bayern, Germany

Oliver Stegle 🆔
German Cancer Research Center
Heidelberg, Germany

ISSN 0302-9743      ISSN 1611-3349 (electronic)
Lecture Notes in Computer Science
ISBN 978-3-031-47678-5      ISBN 978-3-031-47679-2 (eBook)
https://doi.org/10.1007/978-3-031-47679-2

This Springer imprint is published by the registered company Springer Nature Switzerland AG
The registered company address is: Gewerbestrasse 11, 6330 Cham, Switzerland

Paper in this product is recyclable.

# Preface

The Workshop on Machine Learning for Multimodal Healthcare Data (ML4MHD 2023) was a pioneering initiative that aimed to bridge the gap between the realms of machine learning and healthcare. Co-located with ICML 2023 in Honolulu, Hawaii, this workshop was a testament to the growing importance of interdisciplinary collaboration. The workshop's primary objective was to bring together experts from diverse fields such as medicine, pathology, biology, and machine learning. These professionals gathered to present novel methods and solutions that address healthcare challenges, especially those that arise from the complexity and heterogeneity of patient data.

The review process for the workshop was rigorous and thorough. A total of 30 full papers were submitted, out of which 18 were accepted. This corresponds to an acceptance rate of 60% and reflects the high standards maintained by the review committee and the quality of the contributions.

The program schedule was a blend of invigorating keynotes and insightful scientific talks. The day began with an opening by the workshop chairs, followed by the first keynote by Fabian Theis on "Learning and using a multimodal single cell atlas." The subsequent presentations covered a wide range of topics, from multimodal fusion in medical imaging to the application of machine learning in predicting disease onset and therapeutic response. Notable keynotes included Marzyeh Ghassemi's exploration of the ethical dimensions of machine learning in health and Judy Wawira's deep dive into the evolution and future trajectory of multimodal AI in radiology. The workshop culminated in a panel discussion, providing a platform for attendees to engage in stimulating debates and discussions.

A standout feature of ML4MHD 2023 is the optional Springer proceedings. This unique offering marries the open-access free publishing ethos of the machine learning community with the medical data processing community's strong desire for published proceedings. These proceedings are now published in the esteemed Lecture Notes of Computer Science series by Springer. Authors were given the flexibility to opt out of the proceedings, reflecting the workshop's commitment to accommodating the diverse preferences of its contributors.

In conclusion, ML4MHD 2023 was a resounding success, fostering a space for knowledge exchange, networking, and collaboration. The workshop's achievements are a testament to the dedication and vision of its organizers and contributors. We, the workshop chairs - Julia A. Schnabel, Andreas K. Maier, Pallavi Tiwari, and Oliver Stegle - extend our heartfelt gratitude to all participants and look forward to future editions of this workshop.

Warm regards,

July 2023

Andreas K. Maier
Julia A. Schnabel
Pallavi Tiwari
Oliver Stegle

# Organization

## General Chairs

Julia A. Schnabel     Technical University of Munich, Germany,
Helmholtz Munich, Germany and King's
College London, UK

Andreas K. Maier     Friedrich-Alexander-Universität
Erlangen-Nürnberg, Germany

Pallavi Tiwari     University of Wisconsin-Madison, USA

Oliver Stegle     German Cancer Research Center, Germany and
European Molecular Biology Laboratory,
Germany

## Program Committee Chairs

Julia A. Schnabel     Technical University of Munich, Germany,
Helmholtz Munich, Germany and King's
College London, UK

Andreas K. Maier     Friedrich-Alexander-Universität
Erlangen-Nürnberg, Germany

Pallavi Tiwari     University of Wisconsin-Madison, USA

Oliver Stegle     German Cancer Research Center, Germany and
European Molecular Biology Laboratory,
Germany

## Scientific Review Committee

Andreas K. Maier     Friedrich-Alexander-Universität
Erlangen-Nürnberg, Germany

Cory McLean     Google, USA

Daniel Lang     Helmholtz Munich, Germany

David Chen     Cleveland Clinic, USA

Dominic Giles     University College London, UK

Erina Ghosh     Philips Research North America, USA

Farhad Hormozdiari     Google, USA

Fuxin Fan     Friedrich-Alexander-Universität
Erlangen-Nürnberg, Germany

| | |
|---|---|
| Hongyi Pan | University of Illinois Chicago, USA |
| Iris Szu-Szu Ho | University of Edinburgh, UK |
| Julia A. Schnabel | Technical University of Munich, Germany, Helmholtz Munich, Germany and King's College London, UK |
| Kai Packhäuser | Friedrich-Alexander-Universität Erlangen-Nürnberg, Germany |
| Karthik Shetty | Friedrich-Alexander-Universität Erlangen-Nürnberg, Germany |
| Kim Branson | GlaxoSmithKline, UK |
| Lee Jeongwon | Korea Advanced Institute of Science and Technology, South Korea |
| Nicholas Furlotte | Google, USA |
| Niharika D'Souza | IBM Research, USA |
| Noah Maul | Friedrich-Alexander-Universität Erlangen-Nürnberg, Germany |
| Parashkev Nachev | University College London, UK |
| Paula Andrea Pérez-Toro | Friedrich-Alexander-Universität Erlangen-Nürnberg, Germany |
| Pedro Sanchez | University of Edinburgh, UK |
| Peter Washington | University of Hawaii at Manoa, USA |
| Ričards Marcinkevičs | ETH Zurich, Switzerland |
| Shohreh Deldari | University of New South Wales, Australia |
| Siming Bayer | Friedrich-Alexander-Universität Erlangen-Nürnberg, Germany |
| Song Wei | Georgia Tech, USA |
| Srikrishna Jaganathan | Friedrich-Alexander-Universität Erlangen-Nürnberg, Germany |
| Tanveer Syeda-Mahmood | IBM Research, USA |
| Tobias Weise | Friedrich-Alexander-Universität Erlangen-Nürnberg, Germany |
| Tomás Arias-Vergara | Friedrich-Alexander-Universität Erlangen-Nürnberg, Germany |
| Vanshali Sharma | IIT Guwahati, India |
| Virginia Fernandez | King's College London |
| Yiqing Shen | Johns Hopkins University, USA |
| Yongsheng Mei | George Washington University, USA |

# Contents

# Death Prediction by Race in Colorectal Cancer Patients Using Machine Learning Approaches

Frances M. Aponte-Caraballo⬤, Frances Heredia-Negrón⬤,
Brenda G. Nieves-Rodriguez, and Abiel Roche-Lima(✉)⬤

CCRHD-RCMI Program, University of Puerto Rico, Medical Sciences Campus, San Juan,
PR 00936, USA
abiel.roche@upr.edu

**Abstract.** Cancer (CRC) cases have increased worldwide. In USA, African Americans have a higher incidence than other races. In this paper, we aimed to use ML to study specific factors or variables affecting the high incidence of CRC mortality by race after receiving treatments and create models to predict death. We used metastatic CRC Genes Sequencing Studies as data. The patient's inclusion was based on receiving chemotherapy and grouped by race (White-American and African-American). Five supervised ML methods were implemented for creating model predictions and a Mini-Batched-Normalized-Mutual-Information-Hybrid-Feature-Selection method to extract features including more than 25,000 genes. As a result, the best model was obtained with the Classification-Regression-Trees algorithm (AUC-ROC = 0.91 for White-American, AUC-ROC = 0.89 for African Americans). The features "DBNL gene", "PIN1P1 gene" and "Days-from-birth" were the most significant variables associated with CRC mortality for White-American, while "IFI44L-gene", "ART4-gene" and "Sex" were the most relevant related to African-American. In conclusion, these features and models are promising for further analysis and decision-making tools to study CRC from a precision medicine perspective for minority health.

**Keywords:** Machine learning · Modelling · Clinical Decision Support · Mortality · Health Disparities

## 1 Introduction

Colorectal Cancer (CRC) cases are increasing worldwide, it is the second most deadly cancer [1, 2]. In USA, African Americans have a higher incidence than other races. For 2020, the Global Cancer Observatory estimated 1.9 million new colorectal cancer cases globally [3]. Ultimately, CRC has been explored as a genetic disease [4]. Over the years, research has made it possible to identify and increase treatment options, targeting specific genes and personalize courses of treatment for patients using machine learning (ML) approaches.

The goal of this work is to study colorectal cancer from a precision medicine perspective using machine learning-based approaches including specific factors or variables

A. K. Maier et al. (Eds.): ML4MHD 2023, LNCS 14315, pp. 1–6, 2024.
https://doi.org/10.1007/978-3-031-47679-2_1

(clinical, sociodemographic, treatment and genes) affecting the high incidence of CRC mortality by race after receiving treatments, as well as creating models to predict death. We used the Metastatic Colorectal Cancer Genes Sequencing Study data from 2018 found in the cBioportal Data Base [4]. We aimed to use ML to identify the most related a-priori variables associated with colorectal cancer mortality after chemotherapy treatments (grouped by race) and created ML-based models to predict death by race using the most related a-priori variables.

## 2    Materials and Methods

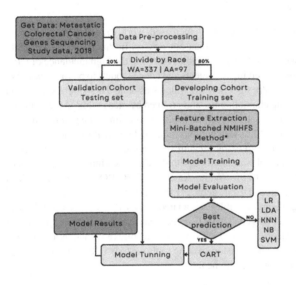

**Fig. 1.** Overview of the methods.

Figure 1 describes the overview of the methods, where First, data is getting from the Metastatic Colorectal Cancer Genes Sequencing Study data from 2018. There were 337 White-Americans (WA) and 97 Africa-Americans (AF). The cohort is divided in Validation (20%) and Training (80%). Several methods were applied to the training set, these were: Feature Extraction, Model Training (with the following ML algorithms - Logistic Regression-LR, Linear Discriminant Analysis-LDA, K-Nearest-Neighbor-KNN, Naive Bayes-NB, Support Vector Machine-SVM and Classification and Regression Tree-CART), Model Evaluation and Model Tuning. Finally, the results were obtained.

## 2.1  Data

The data for this study was obtained from the Metastatic Colorectal Cancer Genes Sequencing Study data, 2018, at cBioportal Data Base [4]. We selected from the database four different files, which are "Patient", "Sample", "Treatment" and "Genes". These files contain different features and samples. A script was developed to merge these files using the "Patient_ID" identifier.

## 2.2  Pre-processing

As a selected criterion, all samples without all the features were removed. In addition, categorical values were converted to dummy variables. As we were interested in patients after getting treatments, all samples instances who received chemotherapy were selected. Then, the dataset was separated by race, obtaining two datasets (1) Whites-American who received chemotherapy (337 patients) and (2) African-Americans who received chemotherapy (97 patients). The independent variable or class was "OS_STATUS" related to death after chemotherapy. This class or variable was selected because we aimed to predict whether the patient died after treatment. Then, these datasets were divided in 80% for training and 20% for testing.

## 2.3  Machine Learning Methods

To identify in the training set the most related features or factors associated with patients' death after treatment, we used the mini-batched Normalized Mutual Information Hybrid Feature Selection (NMIHFS) method developed by Thejas and collaborators, 2019 [5]. This feature selection method improves computational efficiency, reducing computational time, and has the capacity to analyze big data sets [5]. This method was used because we considered all the values for gene expression that totalized more than 25,000 independent features, along with other clinical and sociodemographic features. Then, NMIHFS method allows to analyze data by batches and being more accurate with feature selection methods.

After the best features were selected, we used these variables to train the ML algorithms for each race group. We used five supervised algorithms, which are Logistic Regression (LR), Linear Discriminant Analysis (LDA), Classification and Regression Tree (CART), K-Nearest-Neighbor (KNN), and Naive-Bayes (NB). As the evaluation metrics, we computed accuracy (ACC) and Area Under the ROC curve (AUC ROC) values for the model obtained by each algorithm.

Then, the best two models (the models with the highest accuracy values) were used to apply the model tuning algorithm. Model tuning algorithms in ML are referred as the procedure to find the best combination of parameters through search methods to optimize the final predictive models [6]. In this case, we used the Grid Search algorithm, which is a parameter tuning technique that attempts to compute the optimum values of each parameter of the algorithm to find the best model results [6]. Grid Search uses all combinations of parameters one by one into the model and check the result, until the best accuracy is obtained. Finally, the best model is obtained and validated with the testing set. Then, this is the proposed model to make future predictions of CRC patients' death after chemotherapy treatment.

## 3   Results and Discussion

For the first dataset, (White-American - 337 samples), the mean age was 59.37 years old with a standard deviation of ±12.11. For the second dataset, (African-American - 97 samples) the mean age was 57.91 with the standard deviation of ±14.31. As a result of the feature extraction, the method successfully identified three important variables associated with death for the White-American dataset, that included two genes (DBNL and PIN1P1) and the "Days to Birth" variable. For the second dataset, African-Americans, four important features were identified, which included 2 genes (IFI44L, ART4), and the two other variables "sex" and "Progress Free Survival (PFS)".

The DBNL, IFI44L and ART4 are important encoding protein, while PIN1P1 is a pseudogene [7–10]. These results imply that expressions values of these genes (over-expressed or under-expressed) are related to death by CRC patients after chemotherapy. Similarly, the sex and the PFS (defined by the National Cancer Institute as the time the patient is living with the disease during or after receiving treatment and the disease do not progress [11]), are relevant for the patients' death.

Regarding the metric values for the trained models, the accuracy results were: (1) White-American dataset, LR (ACC = 0.85), LDA (ACC = 0.86), CART (ACC = 0.95), KNN (ACC = 0.86) and NB (ACC = 0.69); (2) African-American dataset, LR (ACC = 0.83), LDA (ACC = 0.84), CART (ACC = 0.97), KNN (ACC = 0.69) and NB (ACC = 0.59). As can be noticed, in both datasets the best model was obtained with the CART algorithm.

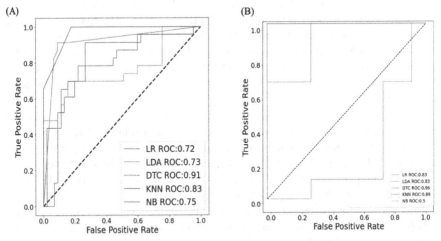

**Fig. 2.** AUC-ROC values for the final models. (A) White-American dataset, (B) African-American dataset

Area Under the ROC Curve values were also computed for each dataset (Fig. 2). Figure 2 (A) shows the values for the White-Americans dataset and Fig. 2 (B) shows the values for African-American dataset. As can be seen, the results are proportional to the ACC values. The obtained models with the CART algorithm had the highest

AUC ROC values (AUC ROC = 0.91 and AUC ROC = 0.96, for White-American and African-American, respectively). These AUC ROC values mean that CART models can distinguish between true and false positives.

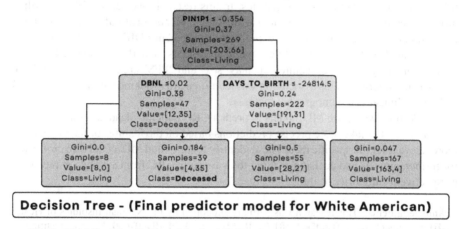

**Decision Tree - (Final predictor model for White American)**

**Fig. 3.** Final Decision Tree model using CART algorithm for White-American dataset.

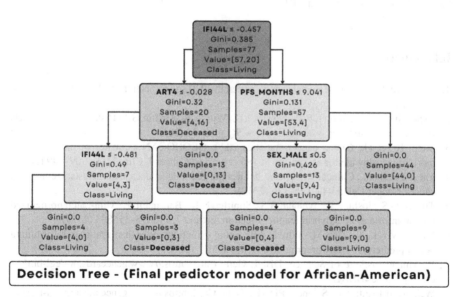

**Decision Tree - (Final predictor model for African-American)**

**Fig. 4.** Final Decision Tree model using CART algorithm for African-American dataset.

Figure 3 and Fig. 4 show the final decision trees obtained with this algorithm to predict death in CRC patients after treatment for White-American and African-American, respectively. Given a new patient's data, these trees can be used to predict if the person is going to die after the chemotherapy is applied.

## 4 Conclusions

Colorectal Cancer increased deaths are a public health problem. Using machine learning approaches for cancer research allows to identify intrinsic ethnic characteristics that are important to understand health disparities. In this research, we successfully identified different features or factors associated with CRC patients' death after chemotherapy, depending on race. In this case, the expressions of the genes DBNL, PIN1P1 and DTB are associated with death for White-American patients, and IFI44L and ART4 gene expression along with other features, such as "sex" and "PFS" are associated with death for African-American. This association was identified after looking among 25,000 genes and other clinical and demographic features.

In addition, we obtain ML models to predict CRC patients' death after treatment by race. It allows to make more precise predictions based on the features or factors that are more relevant for the specific race. These identify features and ML models are promising for further analysis and decision-making tools to study CRC from a precision medicine perspective for minority health.

**Acknowledgments.** This research was partially supported by the National Institutes of Health (NIH) Agreement NO. 1OT2OD032581-01; RCMI grants U54 MD007600 (National Institute on Minority Health and Health Disparities) from NIH; and CAPAC Grant Number R25CA240120 (National Cancer Institute) from NIH.

## References

1. Xi, Y., Xu, P.: Global colorectal cancer burden in 2020 and projections to 2040. Transl. Oncol. **14** (2021)
2. Usher-Smith, J.A., Walter, F.M., Emery, J.D., Win, A.K., Griffin, S.J.: Risk prediction models for colorectal cancer: a systematic review **9**(1), 13–26 (2016)
3. Sung, H., et al.: Global cancer statistics 2020: GLOBOCAN estimates of incidence and mortality worldwide for 36 cancers in 185 countries. Cancer J. Clin. **71**(3), 209–249 (2021)
4. Yaeger, R., et al.: Clinical sequencing defines the genomic landscape of metastatic colorectal cancer. Cancer Cell **33**(1), 125–136 (2018)
5. Thejas, G.S., Joshi, S.R., Iyengar, S.S., Sunitha, N.R., Badrinath, P.: Mini-batch normalized mutual information: a hybrid feature selection method **7**, 116875–116885 (2019)
6. Fu, W., Vivek, N., Tim, M.: Why is differential evolution better than grid search for tuning defect predictors? arXiv preprint arXiv:1609.02613 (2016)
7. Weizmann Institute of Science: DBNL Gene Card. https://www.genecards.org/cgi-bin/car ddisp.pl?gene=DBNL
8. Weizmann Institute of Science: PIN1P1 Gene Card. https://www.genecards.org/cgi-bin/car ddisp.pl?gene=PIN1P1
9. Weizmann Institute of Science: IFI44L Gene Card. https://www.genecards.org/cgi-bin/car ddisp.pl?gene=IFI44L
10. Weizmann Institute of Science: ART 4 Gene Card. https://www.genecards.org/cgi-bin/car ddisp.pl?gene=ART4
11. National Cancer Institute: Progression-Free Survival. https://www.cancer.gov/publications/ dictionaries/cancer-terms/def/progression-free-survival

# Neural Graph Revealers

Harsh Shrivastava$^{(\boxtimes)}$ and Urszula Chajewska

Microsoft Research, Redmond, USA
{hshrivastava,urszc}@microsoft.com

**Abstract.** Sparse graph recovery methods work well where the data follows their assumptions, however, they are not always designed for doing downstream probabilistic queries. This limits their adoption to only identifying connections among domain variables. On the other hand, Probabilistic Graphical Models (PGMs) learn an underlying base graph together with a distribution over the variables (nodes). PGM design choices are carefully made such that the inference and sampling algorithms are efficient. This results in certain restrictions and simplifying assumptions. In this work, we propose Neural Graph Revealers (NGRs) which attempt to efficiently merge the sparse graph recovery methods with PGMs into a single flow. The task is to recover a sparse graph showing connections between the features and learn a probability distribution over them at the same time. NGRs use a neural network as a multitask learning framework. We introduce *graph-constrained path norm* that NGRs leverage to learn a graphical model that captures complex non-linear functional dependencies between features in the form of an undirected sparse graph. NGRs can handle multimodal inputs like images, text, categorical data, embeddings etc. which are not straightforward to incorporate in the existing methods. We show experimental results on data from Gaussian graphical models and a multimodal infant mortality dataset by CDC (Software: https://github.com/harshs27/neural-graph-revealers).

**Keywords:** Sparse Graph Recovery · Probabilistic Graphical Models · Deep Learning

## 1 Introduction

Sparse graph recovery is an important tool to gain insights from data and a widely researched topic [18,32,35]. Given an input data $X$ with $M$ samples and $D$ features, the graph recovery algorithms discover feature dependencies in the form of a sparse graph, $S_g \in \mathbb{R}^{D \times D}$, where $S_g$ is the adjacency matrix. Such graphs are useful for analyzing data from various domains, for instance, obtaining gene regulatory networks from single-cell RNA sequencing data [16,25,43,44]. In the finance domain, a graph showing correspondence between various companies can be obtained using the stock market data. Similarly, understanding automobile sensor networks for navigation purposes [15]. Other interesting applications

© The Author(s), under exclusive license to Springer Nature Switzerland AG 2024
A. K. Maier et al. (Eds.): ML4MHD 2023, LNCS 14315, pp. 7–25, 2024.
https://doi.org/10.1007/978-3-031-47679-2_2

consist of studying brain connectivity patterns in autistic patients [27], increasing methane yield in the anaerobic digestion process [37,38], gaining insights from the infant-mortality data by CDC [36] and multivariate timeseries segmentation [20]. These sparse graphs can be directed, undirected or have mixed-edge types.

The space of graph recovery algorithms is quite substantial (see Fig. 1), so to narrow down the scope of exploration, we only consider the problem of recovering undirected graphs in this work. Ideally, an algorithm for sparse graph recovery should have the following properties: (I) Have a rich functional representation to capture complex functional dependencies among features, (II) Handle diverse data types within the same framework, (III) Enforce sparsity, (IV) Run unsupervised as acquiring ground truth data can be expensive or impossible, (V) Be efficient and scalable to handle large number of features.

It is a difficult to design methods that can achieve a good balance between the desiderata mentioned. Many existing approaches make simplifying assumptions about the distribution in order to achieve sparsity [3,11,16,25,48]. Some use the deep unfolding technique to use the existing optimization algorithm as an inductive bias for designing deep learning architectures [33,34]. These deep unfolding based methods can achieve scalability and sparsity at the cost of making assumptions about the underlying joint probability distribution [27,38,39] and require supervision for learning.

In this work, we present an efficient algorithm, called Neural Graph Revealers (NGRs), that aspires to achieve the optimum balance between the listed desiderata. NGRs can model highly non-linear and complex functional dependencies between features by leveraging the expressive power of neural networks. It is a regression based approach that takes the $D$ features as input and maps them to the same features as the output. In order to achieve sparsity without compromising on the function representation capacity, NGRs leverage the idea of viewing the neural networks as a *glass box*, with model architecture encoding domain insights in a way that can be easily accessed. The NNs can be considered a multitask learning framework The paths between the input and output units are used to capture feature dependencies and thus restricting these paths (eg. using path-norms) can enforce desired sparsity in an unsupervised manner. Thus, NGRs recover undirected graphs that reveal the functional dependencies between the features. Furthermore, the design of NGRs adhere to a special type of probabilistic graphical models known as Neural Graphical Models [36]. Thus, after learning the NGR parameters, one can also query them for probabilistic reasoning, inference and sampling tasks.

Key features and contributions of this work are:

- Novel use of neural networks as a multi-task learning framework to model functional dependencies jointly for all features that enables richer and more complex representation as compared to the state-of-the-art methods.
- Incorporating multi-modal feature types like images, text, categorical data or generic embeddings.

– Training is unsupervised which facilitates wider applicability and adoption to
  new domains.
– Scalable approach to handle a large number of features.
– Once learned, the NGR architecture becomes an instance of a Neural Graphical
  Model and can be used for downstream probabilistic reasoning tasks.

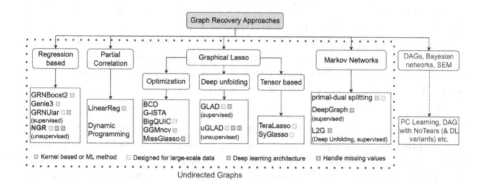

**Fig. 1. Graph Recovery approaches.** Methods designed to recover undirected
graphs are categorized. Neural Graph Revealers (NGRs ) are listed under the regression based algorithms. The algorithms (leaf nodes) listed here are representative of the
sub-category and the list is not exhaustive (Figure borrowed from [35]).

## 2   Related Methods

Figure 1 is an attempt to categorize different methods to recover graphs. Broadly
speaking, we can divide them into approaches recovering directed graphs and
the ones recovering undirected or mixed-edge graphs. In this work, we primarily
focus on methods developed for undirected graphs. Directed graphs have different
semantics, with more complex dependence ralationships encoded by edges. They
are sometimes used to determine causality [26]. Bayesian network graphs can
be converted to their undirected versions by the process of moralization [21].
We focus on modeling pairwise dependencies and not causation in this work, so
undirected graphs will suffice. For the purpose of categorizing different methods
that recover undirected graphs, we break-down methods into the ones based on
solving the graphical lasso objective also known as Conditional Independence
(CI) graphs, the ones directly evaluating partial correlations, and the ones based
on the regression formulation. The remaining methods are under the Markov
networks umbrella.

*Regression Based Approaches.* Consider the input data $X \in \mathbb{R}^{M \times D}$ with $D$
features and $M$ samples. For each of the $D$ features, the regression based
formulation fits a regression function with respect to all the other features,

$X_d = f_d(X_{\{D\}\setminus d}) + \epsilon$, where $\epsilon$ is an additive noise term. After fitting the regression, based on the choice of functions $f'_d s$, the algorithms determine the dependency of the features. These approaches have been very successful for the task of recovering Gene Regulatory Networks. For instance, GENIE3 [48] modeled each $f_d$ to be random forest model while TIGRESS [16] chose linear functions and GRNBoost2 [25] combined random forests with gradient boosting technique to achieve superior performance among others [1,24,31,51]. Then, neural network based representation like GRNUlar [43,44] were developed, which utilized the idea of using NNs as a multitask learning setup. This method is architecturally quite close to our formulation, although the major difference with NGRs is that GRNUlar needs supervision for training. The proposed NGR method can be categorized as a regression based approach. Unlike most other approaches in this group, it can model features that are not real-valued.

*Graphical Lasso Formulation.* Sparse graph recovery based on the graphical lasso formulation and its variants have been extensively studied; a recent survey [35] provides a good primer into these approaches. The traditional optimization based algorithms like BCD [2], G-ISTA [30], BigQUIC [19], GGMncv [50], MissGlasso [46] have been designed to meet a range of requirements like scaling to a large number of features, handling missing values, including non-convex penalties etc. The TeraLasso [14] and the Sylvester Graphical Lasso or SyGlasso model [49] are tensor based approaches and have recently garnered more interest. The methods in this category assume a multivariate Gaussian as the underlying distribution which might not be suitable for certain problems. The deep unfolding based approaches have been shown to capture tail distributions and demonstrate better sample complexity results. GLAD [39] and its unsupervised version uGLAD [37], can perform competitively with the existing approaches.

*Partial Correlation Evaluation.* Methods belonging to this category aim to directly calculate partial correlations between all pairs of features to determine the Conditional Independence (CI) graph between the features. Algorithms based on fitting linear regression or using dynamic programming to evaluate the partial correlation formula directly have been developed [35].

*Markov Networks.* Probabilistic Graphical Models defined over undirected graphs are known as Markov Networks (MNs). Structure learning of MNs has been discussed extensively in [13,21,22,35]. Some of the recent deep learning based methods can capture rich functional dependencies like DeepGraph [3], which uses convolutional neural networks to learn graph structure and L2G [27] that uses the deep unfolding technique to convert optimization algorithm templates into a deep architecture. Though these methods are interesting and improve upon their predecessors, they require supervision for training which hinders their wider adoption.

*Directed Graph Recovery Approaches.* Bayesian Networks and causal models like Structural Equation models are represented using directed acyclic graphs (DAGs) [21,26]. The structure learning problem of Bayesian Networks is NP-complete [8], so often heuristic-based algorithms are proposed [45]. Since our work focuses on recovering undirected graphs, we use this opportunity to draw out some similarities between NGRs and the methods developed for DAG recovery. In a recent work, "DAGs with NO TEARS" [54], the authors converted the combinatorial optimization problem into a continuous one and provided an associated optimization algorithm to recover sparse DAGs. This eventually spawned research that provided improvements and also captured complex functional dependencies by introducing deep learning variants [52,53]. One such follow up work [55] we found to be the close to our method in terms of function representation capacity, specifically the MLP version of the nonparametric DAG learning. It uses a separate neural network for modeling each functional dependency of the graph. Although this leads to performance improvements, it also results in having a large number of learnable parameters as compared to NGRs that model all the complex dependencies using a single NN by leveraging the multitask learning framework. In addition, a separate regression model for each feature may lead to inconsistencies in the learned distribution [17].

## 3    Neural Graph Revealers

We assume we are given the input data $X$ with D features and M samples. The task is to recover a sparse graph represented by its adjacency matrix $S_g \in \mathbb{R}^{D \times D}$. In the recovered undirected graph obtained by a regression based approach, each feature or graph node is a function of its immediate (one-hop) neighbors, as shown in Fig. 2(right). In this section, we describe our proposed NGRs along with potential extensions.

### 3.1    Representation

We choose a multilayer perceptron (MLP) as our neural network choice. The architecture of an NGR model is an MLP that takes in input features and fits a regression to get the same features as the output, shown in Fig. 2(left). We start with a fully connected network. Some edges are dropped during training. We view the trained neural network as a glass-box where a path to an output unit (or neuron) from a set of input units means that the output unit is a function of those input units.

In order to obtain a graph, for every feature $X_d$, we want to find the most relevant features that have a direct functional influence on $X_d$. This task becomes increasingly complex as we need to evaluate all possible combinations which can be computationally tedious. Fitting the regression of NGRs, refer to Fig. 2(middle), can be seen as doing *multitask learning* that simultaneously optimizes for the functional dependencies of all the features.

Main design challenges in fitting the NGR regression are:

(A) How do we avoid modeling direct self-dependencies among features, eg. $X_d \rightarrow X_d, \forall d \in \{D\}$?

(B) How do we efficiently induce sparsity among the paths defined by the MLP?

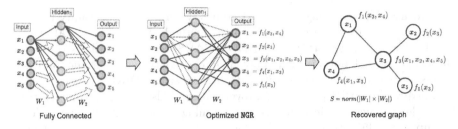

**Fig. 2.** *Workflow of NGRs.* (left) We start with a fully connected Neural Network (MLP here) where both the input and the output represent the given features $x_i's$. Viewing NN as a multitask learning framework indicates that the output features are dependent on all the input features in the initial fully connected setting. (middle) The learned NGR optimizes the network connections to fit the regression on the input data as well as satisfy the sparsity constraints, refer to Eq. 2. A presence of a path from the input feature to an output feature indicates a dependency, potentially non-linear, between them. The bigger the size of NN (number of layers, hidden unit dimensions) the richer will be the functional representation. Note that not all the weights of the MLP (those dropped during training in grey-dashed lines) are shown for the sake of clarity. (right) The sparse dependency graph between the input and the output of the MLP reduces to the normalized weight matrix product $S_g = \text{norm}\left(|W_1| \times |W_2|\right)$.

### 3.2   Optimization

We denote a NN with $L$ number of layers with the weights $\mathcal{W} = \{W_1, W_2, \cdots, W_L\}$ and biases $\mathcal{B} = \{b_1, b_2, \cdots, b_L\}$ as $f_{\mathcal{W},\mathcal{B}}(\cdot)$ with non-linearity not mentioned explicitly. In our implementation, we experimented with multiple non-linearities and found that ReLU fits well with our framework. Applying the NN to the input $X$ evaluates the following mathematical expression, $f_{\mathcal{W},\mathcal{B}}(X) = \text{ReLU}(W_L \cdot (\cdots (W_2 \cdot \text{ReLU}(W_1 \cdot X + b_1) + b_2) \cdots) + b_L)$. The dimensions of the weights and biases are chosen such that the neural network input and output units are equal to $\mathcal{D}$ while the hidden layers dimension $H$ remains a design choice. In our experiments, we found a good initial choice of $H = 2|\mathcal{D}|$. It can be adjusted based on the loss on validation data.

Our task is to design the NGR objective function such that it can jointly discover the feature dependency graph constraints (A) & (B) along with fitting the regression on the input data. We observe that the product of the weights of the neural network $S_{nn} = \prod_{l=1}^{L} |W_l| = |W_1| \times |W_2| \times \cdots \times |W_L|$, where $|W|$ computes the absolute value of each element in $W$, gives us path dependencies between the input and the output units. We note that if $S_{nn}[x_i, x_o] = 0$ then the output unit $x_o$ does not depend on input unit $x_i$.

**Graph-Constrained Path Norm.** We introduce a way to map NN paths to a predefined graph structure. Consider the matrix $S_{nn}$ that maps the paths from the input units to the output units as described above. Assume we are given a graph with adjacency matrix $S_g \in \{0,1\}^{D \times D}$. The graph-constrained path norm is defined as $\mathcal{P}_c = \left\| S_{nn} * S_g^c \right\|_1$, where $S_g^c$ is the complement of the adjacency matrix $S_g^c = J_D - S_g$ with $J_D \in \{1\}^{D \times D}$ being an all-ones matrix. The operation $Q * V$ represents the Hadamard operator which does an element-wise matrix multiplication between the same dimension matrices $Q$ & $V$. This term is used to enforce penalty to fit a particular predefined graph structure, $S_g$.

We use this formulation of MLPs to model the constraints along with finding the set of parameters $\{\mathcal{W}, \mathcal{B}\}$ that minimize the regression loss expressed as the Euclidean distance between $X$ and $f_{\mathcal{W},\mathcal{B}}(X)$. Optimization becomes

$$\arg\min_{\mathcal{W},\mathcal{B}} \sum_{k=1}^{M} \left\| X^k - f_{\mathcal{W},\mathcal{B}}(X^k) \right\|_2^2 \quad s.t. \quad \mathrm{sym}(S_{nn}) * S_{\mathrm{diag}} = 0 \qquad (1)$$

where, $\mathrm{sym}(S_{nn}) = \left( \|S_{nn}\|_2 + \|S_{nn}\|_2^T \right)/2$ converts the path norm obtained by the NN weights product, $S_{nn} = \prod_{l=1}^{L} |W_l|$, into a symmetric adjacency matrix and $S_{\mathrm{diag}} \in \mathbb{R}^{D \times D}$ represents a matrix of zeroes except the diagonal entries that are 1. Constraint (A) is thus included as the constraint term in Eq. 1. To satisfy the constraint (B), we include an $\ell_1$ norm term $\|\mathrm{sym}(S_{nn})\|_1$ which will introduce sparsity in the path norms. Note that this second constraint enforces sparsity of *paths*, not individual *weights*, thus affecting the entire network structure.

We model these constraints as Lagrangian terms which are scaled by a log function. The log scaling is done for computational reasons as sometimes the values of the Lagrangian terms can go very low. The constants $\lambda, \gamma$ act as a tradeoff between fitting the regression term and satisfying the corresponding constraints. The optimization formulation to recover a valid graph structure becomes

$$\arg\min_{\mathcal{W},\mathcal{B}} \sum_{k=1}^{M} \left\| X^k - f_{\mathcal{W},\mathcal{B}}(X^k) \right\|_2^2 + \lambda \left\| \mathrm{sym}(S_{nn}) * S_{\mathrm{diag}} \right\|_1 + \gamma \left\| \mathrm{sym}(S_{nn}) \right\|_1 \quad (2)$$

where we can optionally add log scaling to the structure constraint terms. Essentially, we start with a fully connected graph and then the Lagrangian terms induce sparsity in the graph. Algorithm 1 describes the procedure to learn the NGR architecture based on optimizing the Eq. 2. We note that the optimization and the graph recovered depend on the choices of the penalty constants $\lambda, \gamma$. Since our loss function contains multiple terms, the loss-balancing technique introduced in [28], can be utilized to get a good initial value of the constants. Then, while running optimization, based on the regression loss value on a held-out validation data, the values of penalty constants can be appropriately chosen.

## 3.3   Modeling Multi-modal Data

It is common to encounter multi-modal data in real-world datasets. For instance, ICU patient records can have information about body vitals (numerical, categorical), nurse notes (natural language) and maybe associated X-rays (images). It will be extremely helpful to get the underlying graph that shows dependencies

---

**Algorithm 1:** Learning NGRs

---

**Function** NGR-training($X$):

 $f_{\mathcal{W}^0} \leftarrow$ Fully connected MLP

 **For** $e = 1, \cdots, E$ **do**

  Xb $\leftarrow X$ (sample a batch)

  $\mathcal{L} = \sum_{k=1}^{M} \left\| \text{Xb}^k - f_{\mathcal{W},\mathcal{B}}(\text{Xb}^k) \right\|^2 - \lambda \left\| \text{sym}(S_{nn}) * S_{\text{diag}} \right\|_1$
  $-\gamma \left\| \text{sym}(S_{nn}) \right\|_1$

  $\mathcal{W}^e, \mathcal{B}^e \leftarrow$ backprop $\mathcal{L}$ with Adam optimizer

 $\{\mathcal{W}^E\} \leftarrow f^E_{\mathcal{W},\mathcal{B}}$

 $\mathcal{G} \leftarrow \text{sym}\left( \prod_{l=1}^{L} |W_l^E| \right)$

 **return** $\mathcal{G}, f_{\mathcal{W}^E}$

---

between these various features. In this section, we propose two different ways to include multi-modal input data in the NGR formulation.

*(I) Using Projection Modules.* Figure 3 gives a schematic view of including projection modules in the base architecture presented in Fig. 2. Without loss of generality, we can assume that each of the $D$ inputs is an embedding in $x_i \in \mathbb{R}^I$ space. For example, given an image, one way of getting a corresponding embedding can be to use the latent layer of a convolutional neural network based autoencoder. We convert all the input $x_i$ nodes in the NGR architecture to hypernodes, where each hypernode contains the embedding vector. Consider a hypernode that contains an embedding vector of size $E$ and if an edge is connected to the hypernode, then that edge is connected to all the $E$ units of the embedding vector. For each of these input hypernodes, we define a corresponding encoder embedding $e_i \leftarrow \text{enc}_i(x_i), \forall e_i \in \mathbb{R}^E$, which can be designed specifically for that particular input embedding. We apply the encoder modules to all the $x_i$ hypernodes and obtain the $e_i$ hypernodes. Same procedure is followed at the decoder end, where $x_i \leftarrow \text{dec}_i(d_i), \forall d_i \in \mathbb{R}^O$. Embeddings are used primarily to reduce input dimensions. The NGR graph discovery optimization reduces to discovering the connectivity pattern using the path norms between hypernodes $e_i$'s and $d_i$'s. A slight modification to the graph-constrained path norm is needed to account for the hypernodes. The $S_{diag}$ term will now represent the connections between the hypernodes, $S_{diag} \in \{0,1\}^{DE \times DO}$ with ones in the block diagonals.

We can include the projection modules in the regression term of the NGR objective, while the structure learning terms will remain intact

$$\underset{\mathcal{W},\mathcal{B},\text{proj}}{\arg\min} \sum_{k=1}^{M} \left\| X^k - f_{\mathcal{W},\mathcal{B},\text{proj}}(X^k) \right\|_2^2 + \lambda \left\| \text{sym}(S_{nn}) * S_{\text{diag}} \right\|_1 + \gamma \left\| \text{sym}(S_{nn}) \right\|_1$$

$$(3)$$

where the proj are the parameters of the encoder and decoder projection modules as shown in Fig. 3.

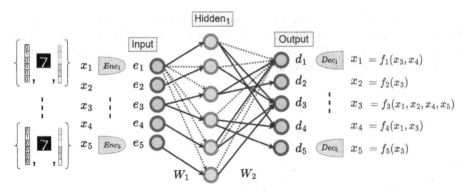

**Fig. 3.** *Multi-modal data handling with projection modules.* The input **X** can be one-hot (categorical), image or in general an embedding (text, audio, speech and other data types). Projection modules (encoder + decoder) are used as a wrapper around the NGR base architecture. The architecture of the projection modules depends on the input data type and users' design choices. Note that the output of the encoder can be more than 1 unit ($e_1$ can be a hypernode) and the corresponding adjacency matrix $S_{\text{diag}}$ of the graph-constrained path norm can be adjusted. Similarly, the decoder side of the NGR architecture is updated. The remaining details are similar to the ones described in Fig. 2.

*(II) Using Graph-Constrained Path Norm (GcPn).* Figure 4 shows that we can view the connections between the $D$ hypernodes of the input embedding $x_i \in \mathbb{R}^I$ (where $I$ is the dimensionality of the input) to the corresponding input of the encoder layer $e_i \in \mathbb{R}^E$ (with $E$ being the dimensionality of the embedding) as a graph. We represent each input layer to the encoder layer connections by $S_{\text{enc}} \in \{0,1\}^{DI \times DE}$, where $S_{\text{enc}}[x_i, e_j] = 1$ if the $(x_i, e_j)$ hypernodes are connected. If we initialize a fully connected neural network (or MLP) between the input layer and the encoder layer, we can utilize the GcPn penalty function to map the paths from the input units to the encoder units to satisfy the graph structure defined by $S_{\text{enc}}$. Similar exercise is replicated at the decoder end to obtain $S_{\text{dec}}$. This extension of the GcPn to multi-modal data leads us to the following Lagrangian based formulation of the optimization objective

$$\underset{\mathcal{W}_{\text{enc}}, \mathcal{W}, \mathcal{B}, \mathcal{W}_{\text{dec}}}{\arg\min} \sum_{k=1}^{M} \left\| X^k - f_{\mathcal{W}_{\text{enc}}, \mathcal{W}, \mathcal{B}, \mathcal{W}_{\text{dec}}}(X^k) \right\|_2^2 + \lambda \left\| \text{sym}(S_{nn}) * S_{\text{diag}} \right\|_1 \quad (4)$$

$$+ \gamma \left\| \text{sym}(S_{nn}) \right\|_1 + \eta \left\| \text{sym}(S_{nn}^e) * S_{\text{enc}} \right\|_1 + \beta \left\| \text{sym}(S_{nn}^d) * S_{\text{dec}} \right\|_1$$

where $f_{\mathcal{W}_{\text{enc}}, \mathcal{W}, \mathcal{B}, \mathcal{W}_{\text{dec}}}(\cdot)$ represents the entire end-to-end MLP including the encoder and decoder mappings, $S_{nn}^e = \prod_{l=1}^{L^e} |W_l| = |W_1| \times |W_2| \times \cdots \times |W_{L^e}|$ captures the path dependencies in the encoder MLP with $L^e$ layers, $S_{nn}^d = \prod_{l=1}^{L^d} |W_l| = |W_1| \times |W_2| \times \cdots \times |W_{L^d}|$ captures the path dependencies in the decoder MLP with $L^d$ layers. The Lagrangian constants $\lambda, \gamma, \eta, \beta$ are initialized in the same manner as outlined in Sect. 3.2. We note the advantage of using the

GcPn penalties to enable **soft enforcing** of the path constraint requirements between the input and output units of the neural networks. We recommend the GcPn based approach (II) as the implementation is straightforward and it is highly scalable and can handle large embedding sizes.

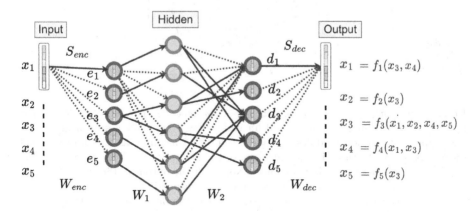

**Fig. 4.** *Multi-modal data handling with graph-constrained path norm.* W.l.o.g. we consider an input **X** to be embeddings that can come from text, audio, speech and other data types. We extend the idea of applying GcPn to the encoder MLP and the decoder MLP. We initialize a fully connected MLP and then using the GcPn penalties, we capture the desired input to output unit path dependencies after optimizing the Eq. 4. Neural network nodes containing embeddings are shown as hypernodes. We use the concept of a hypernode to convey that all units of the embedding vector within the hypernode are considered a single unit when deciding the edge connections defining a graph. The encoder and decoder MLPs are used as a wrapper around the NGR base architecture. The remaining details are similar to the ones described in Fig. 2.

### 3.4   Representation as a Probabilistic Graphical Model

Once the sparse graph is recovered, the learned architecture of NGR represents functional dependencies between the features. In addition, the resulting network has the ability to model the entire joint probability distribution of the features. This type of representation of the functional dependencies based on neural networks has been recently explored in [36] and is called a Neural Graphical Model (NGM). It is a type of a Probabilistic Graphical Model that utilizes neural networks and a pre-defined graph structure between features to learn complex non-linear underlying distributions. Additionally, it can model multi-modal data and has efficient inference and sampling algorithms. The inference capability can be used to estimate missing values in data. The learned NGR model can be viewed as an instance of an NGM.

## 4   Experiments

### 4.1   Learning Gaussian Graphical Models

We explored the NGR's ability to model Gaussian Graphical Models (GGM). To create a GGM, we used a chain-graph structure and then defined a precision matrix over it by randomly initializing the entries $\mathcal{U}(0.5, 1)$ with random signs. The diagonal entries of the precision matrix were chosen such that it is positive semi-definite. Samples were obtained from the GGM and were used as input to the NGR for recovering the underlying graphical model. Figure 5 shows the GGM and the corresponding trends discovered after fitting a NGR. We used a NGR with a single hidden layer with dimension $H = 100$. Table 1 shows the graph recovery results by running NGR on varying number of samples obtained using the Gaussian graphical model. As expected, the results improve as we increase the number of samples and thereby we conclude that NGRs are capable of representing Gaussian graphical models.

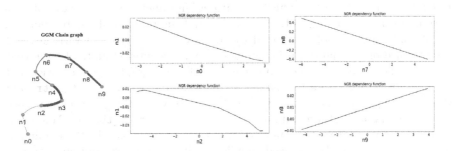

**Fig. 5.** *Modeling GGMs using NGRs.* (left) The Conditional Independence graph [35] for the chain structure used to generate the data. Positive partial correlations between the nodes are shown in green, while the negative partial correlations in red. A positive partial correlation between nodes (A, B) will mean that increasing the value of A will correspond to an increase in value of B. Partial negative correlation will mean the opposite. These correlations show direct dependence or, in other words, the dependence is evaluated conditioned on all the other nodes. (middle, right) Pairwise dependence functions learned by the NGR. We observe that the NGR slopes match the trend in the GGM graph. This shows that the dependency plots learned comply with the desired behaviour as shown in the color of the partial correlation edges. (Color figure online)

### 4.2   Infant Mortality Data Analysis

The infant mortality dataset we used is based on CDC Birth Cohort Linked Birth - Infant Death Data Files [47]. It describes pregnancy and birth variables for all live births in the U.S. together with an indication of an infant's death (and its cause) before the first birthday. We used the latest available dataset, which includes information about 3,988,733 live births in the US during 2015.

**Table 1.** The recovered CI graph from NGR is compared with the ground truth CI graph defined by the underlying GGMs precision matrix with $D = 10$ nodes, chain graph as shown in Fig. 5. Area under the ROC curve (AUC) and area under the precision-recall curve (AUPR) values for 5 runs are reported.

| Samples | AUPR | AUC |
|---|---|---|
| 100 | $0.34 \pm 0.03$ | $0.67 \pm 0.05$ |
| 500 | $0.45 \pm 0.10$ | $0.79 \pm 0.03$ |
| 1000 | $0.63 \pm 0.11$ | $0.90 \pm 0.03$ |

We recoded various causes of death into 12 classes: alive, top 10 distinct causes of death, and death due to other causes.

*Recovered Graphs.* We recovered the graph structure of the dataset using NGR, uGLAD [38] and using Bayesian network package bnlearn [32] with Tabu search and AIC score. The graphs are shown in Fig. 6. All variables were converted to categorical for bnlearn structure learning and inference as it does not support networks containing both continuous and discrete variables. In contrast, uGLAD and NGRs are both equipped to work with mixed types of variables and were trained on the dataset prior to conversion. It is interesting to observe that although there are some common clusters in all three graphs (parents' race and ethnicity (mrace & frace); variables related to mother's bmi, height (mhtr) and weight, both pre-pregnancy (pwgt_r) and at delivery (dwgt_r); type of insurance (pay); parents' ages (fage and mage variables); birth order (tbo and lbo) etc.), each graph has a different extent of inter-cluster connections. The three different graph recovery methods are based on different distribution assumptions, training methodology, way of handling multimodal data, which leads to different connectivity patterns. This dataset and corresponding BN and uGLAD graphs analysis are discussed in [36].

**Table 2.** Comparison of predictive accuracy for gestational age and birthweight.

| Methods | Gestational age (ordinal, weeks) | | Birthweight (continuous, grams) | |
|---|---|---|---|---|
| | MAE | RMSE | MAE | RMSE |
| Logistic Regression | $1.512 \pm 0.005$ | $3.295 \pm 0.043$ | N/A | N/A |
| Bayesian network | $\mathbf{1.040 \pm 0.003}$ | $2.656 \pm 0.027$ | N/A | N/A |
| EBM | $1.313 \pm 0.002$ | $2.376 \pm 0.021$ | $\mathbf{345.21 \pm 1.47}$ | $\mathbf{451.59 \pm 2.38}$ |
| NGM w/full graph | $1.560 \pm 0.067$ | $2.681 \pm 0.047$ | $394.90 \pm 11.25$ | $517.24 \pm 11.51$ |
| NGM w/BN graph | $1.364 \pm 0.025$ | $2.452 \pm 0.026$ | $370.20 \pm 1.44$ | $484.82 \pm 1.88$ |
| NGM w/uGLAD graph | $1.295 \pm 0.010$ | $\mathbf{2.370 \pm 0.025}$ | $371.27 \pm 1.78$ | $485.39 \pm 1.86$ |
| NGR | $1.448 \pm 0.133$ | $2.493 \pm 0.100$ | $369.68 \pm 1.14$ | $483.96 \pm 1.56$ |

**Table 3.** Comparison of predictive accuracy for 1-year survival and cause of death. Note: recall set to zero when there are no labels of a given class, and precision set to zero when there are no predictions of a given class.

| Methods | Survival (binary) | | Cause of death (multivalued, majority class frequency 0.9948) | | | |
|---|---|---|---|---|---|---|
| | AUC | AUPR | micro-averaged | | macro-averaged | |
| | | | Precision | Recall | Precision | Recall |
| Logistic Regression | $0.633 \pm 0.004$ | $0.182 \pm 0.008$ | $0.995 \pm 7.102e{-}05$ | $0.995 \pm 7.102e{-}05$ | $0.136 \pm 0.011$ | $0.130 \pm 0.002$ |
| Bayesian network | $0.655 \pm 0.004$ | $0.252 \pm 0.007$ | $0.995 \pm 7.370e{-}05$ | $0.995 \pm 7.370e{-}05$ | $0.191 \pm 0.008$ | $0.158 \pm 0.002$ |
| EBM | $0.680 \pm 0.003$ | $\mathbf{0.299 \pm 0.007}$ | $0.995 \pm 5.371e{-}05$ | $0.995 \pm 5.371e{-}05$ | $0.228 \pm 0.014$ | $0.166 \pm 0.002$ |
| NGM w/full graph | $0.721 \pm 0.024$ | $0.197 \pm 0.014$ | $0.994 \pm 1.400e{-}05$ | $0.994 \pm 1.400e{-}05$ | $0.497 \pm 7.011e{-}06$ | $\mathbf{0.500 \pm 1.000e{-}06}$ |
| NGM w/BN graph | $0.752 \pm 0.012$ | $0.295 \pm 0.010$ | $0.995 \pm 4.416e{-}05$ | $0.995 \pm 4.416e{-}05$ | $0.497 \pm 2.208e{-}05$ | $\mathbf{0.500 \pm 1.000e{-}06}$ |
| NGM w/uGLAD graph | $0.726 \pm 0.020$ | $0.269 \pm 0.018$ | $0.995 \pm 9.735e{-}05$ | $0.995 \pm 9.735e{-}05$ | $0.497 \pm 4.868e{-}05$ | $\mathbf{0.500 \pm 1.000e{-}06}$ |

*NGR Architecture Details.* Since we have mixed input data types, real and categorical data, we utilize the NGR multimodal architecture's neural view given in Fig. 4. We used a 2-layer neural view with $H = 1000$. The categorical input was converted to its one-hot vector representation and added to the real features which gave us roughly $\sim$500 features as input.

Same dimension settings were replicated at the decoder end. NGR was trained on the 4 million data points with $D = 500$ using 64 CPUs within 4 h.

*Inference Accuracy Comparison.* Infant mortality dataset is particularly challenging due to the data skewness. For instance, the cases of infant death during the first year of life are rare compared to cases of surviving infants. Getting good performance on imbalanced data is a challenging problem and multiple techniques have been developed to assist existing learning algorithms [4,7,41]. We do not report results on applying these techniques as it would be out of scope for this work. Since NGR becomes an instance of a Neural Graphical Model, we also include comparisons of NGMs that use base graphs obtained from Bayesian network, CI graph from uGLAD and also show the results on using a fully connected graph which basically avoids using any internal graph structure. We compared prediction for four variables of various types: gestational age (ordinal, expressed in weeks), birthweight (continuous, specified in grams), survival till 1st birthday (binary) and cause of death ('alive', 10 most common causes of death with less common grouped in category 'other' with 'alive' indicated for 99.48% of infants). We compared with other prediction methods like logistic regression, Bayesian networks, Explainable Boosting Machines (EBM) [6,23] and report 5-fold cross validation results.

Tables 2 and 3 demonstrate that NGR models are more accurate than logistic regression, Bayesian Networks and on par with EBM models for categorical and ordinal variables. Their performance is similar to the NGM models with different input base graphs highlighting that learning a NGR graph can help us gain new insights. We note an additional advantage of NGRs and NGMs in general: we just need to train a single model and their inference capability can be leveraged to output predictions for the multiple tasks listed here. In the case of EBM and LR models, we had to train a separate model for each outcome variable evaluated.

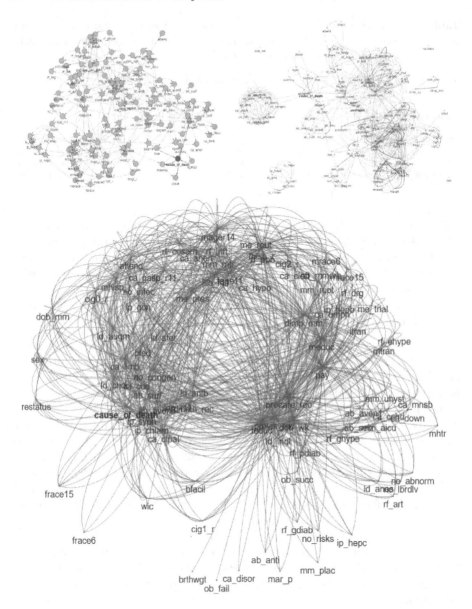

**Fig. 6.** *Graphs recovered for the Infant Mortality 2015 data.* (top left) The Bayesian network graph learned using score-based method, (top right) the CI graph recovered by uGLAD and (bottom) the NGR graph. For NGR, we applied a threshold to retain top relevant edges.

# 5    Conclusions, Discussion and Future Work

We address the important problem of performing sparse graph recovery and querying the corresponding graphical model. The existing graph recovery algorithms make simplifying assumptions about the feature dependency functions in order to achieve sparsity. Some deep learning based algorithms achieve non-linear functional dependencies but their architecture demands too many learnable parameters. After obtaining the underlying graph representation, running probabilistic inference on such models is often unclear and complicated. Neural Graph Revealers leverage neural networks as a multitask learning framework to represent complex distributions and also introduce the concept of graph-constrained path norm to learn a sparse graphical model. The model is an instance of a special type of neural networks based PGMs known as Neural Graphical Models that have efficient algorithms for downstream reasoning tasks. Experiments on infant mortality show the ability of NGRs to model complex multimodal real-world problems.

**Effects of Class Imbalance in Data on Graph Recovery:** In our experiments, we found that the graphs recovered are sensitive to class imbalance. We found that **none** of the prior graph recovery methods identify this issue. The NGR architecture provides flexibility in handling such class imbalanced data. We can leverage the existing data augmentation techniques [7,9] or cost function balancing techniques between data points belonging to different classes [4,5,41,42]. The sparsity induced in the NNs by GcPn makes the NGRs robust to noisy data and makes it a potential candidate to handle imbalance as indicated by its superior performance on predicting cause of death in the infant mortality dataset (Table 3).

**Utilizing Graph Connections for Randomized Neural Networks:** The research on sparse graph recovery along with the associated graphical model obtained using Neural Graph Revealers opens up a possibility of finding connections with the theory of randomized neural networks [10,12,29,40].

We believe that this direction of research can lead to a wider adoption of sparse graph recovery methods as the resulting PGM obtained from NGR has powerful representation and inference capability.

# 6    NGR Design Choices

We share the design choices tried for NGRs that led to the architecture presented in this paper in order to increase transparency and adoption.

- The structure enforcing terms like $\|\text{sym}(S_{nn}) * S_{\text{diag}}\|$ , $\|\text{sym}(S_{nn})\|$ were tried. This included applying $\ell_1$ norm, Frobenius norm and higher order norms. We also found the nonzero counts of dependency matrices to be effective.
- We optionally tried enforcing symmetry of the output $S_{nn}$ or the adjacency matrix by adding a soft threshold term $\left\|S_{nn} - S_{nn}^T\right\|$ with various norms.

– Optimization is tricky due to the multiple loss terms in the objective function. We found that training NGRs can be sensitive to the hyperparameter choices like learning rate, optimizer choice (we primarily used Adam) and the hidden layer dimension. The choice of $\lambda$, which balances between the regression loss and the structure losses is tricky to decide. When optimizing NGR, we observe that it first optimizes the regression loss, then when the regression loss stabilizes, the structure loss gets optimized which increases the regression loss a bit and then eventually both losses go down smoothly. Our general approach to train NGRs is to choose a large number of training epochs with low learning rates. Optionally, log scaling of the structure penalty terms help in stabilizing convergence.

## Ethical Concerns

Our method does not introduce any new ethical issues, however, ethical considerations would be of utmost importance if it were to be applied to sensitive data. Anonymized infant mortality data is meant to generate insights into risk factors, primarily for use by doctors. It is not intended to offer medical advice to expecting parents.

## References

1. Aluru, M., Shrivastava, H., Chockalingam, S.P., Shivakumar, S., Aluru, S.: EnGRaiN: a supervised ensemble learning method for recovery of large-scale gene regulatory networks. Bioinformatics **38**, 1312–1319 (2021)
2. Banerjee, O., Ghaoui, L.E., d'Aspremont, A.: Model selection through sparse maximum likelihood estimation for multivariate Gaussian or binary data. J. Mach. Learn. Rese. **9**, 485–516 (2008)
3. Belilovsky, E., Kastner, K., Varoquaux, G., Blaschko, M.B.: Learning to discover sparse graphical models. In: International Conference on Machine Learning, pp. 440–448. PMLR (2017)
4. Bhattacharya, S., Rajan, V., Shrivastava, H.: ICU mortality prediction: a classification algorithm for imbalanced datasets. In: Proceedings of the AAAI Conference on Artificial Intelligence, vol. 31 (2017)
5. Bhattacharya, S., Rajan, V., Shrivastava, H.: Methods and systems for predicting mortality of a patient, US Patent 10,463,312, 5 November 2019
6. Caruana, R., Lou, Y., Gehrke, J., Koch, P., Sturm, M., Elhadad, N.: Intelligible models for healthcare: predicting pneumonia risk and hospital 30-day readmission. In: Proceedings of the 21th ACM SIGKDD International Conference on Knowledge Discovery and Data Mining, pp. 1721–1730. ACM (2015)
7. Chawla, N.V., Bowyer, K.W., Hall, L.O., Kegelmeyer, W.P.: SMOTE: synthetic minority over-sampling technique. J. Artif. Intell. Res. **16**, 321–357 (2002)
8. Chickering, D.M.: Learning Bayesian networks is NP-complete. In: Fisher, D., Lenz, HJ. (eds.) Learning from Data. Lecture Notes in Statistics, vol. 112, pp. 121–130. Springer, New York (1996). https://doi.org/10.1007/978-1-4612-2404-4_12
9. Fernández, A., Garcia, S., Herrera, F., Chawla, N.V.: SMOTE for learning from imbalanced data: progress and challenges, marking the 15-year anniversary. J. Artif. Intell. Res. **61**, 863–905 (2018)

10. Frankle, J., Carbin, M.: The lottery ticket hypothesis: finding sparse, trainable neural networks. arXiv preprint arXiv:1803.03635 (2018)

11. Friedman, J., Hastie, T., Tibshirani, R.: Sparse inverse covariance estimation with the graphical lasso. Biostatistics **9**(3), 432–441 (2008)

12. Gallicchio, C., Scardapane, S.: Deep randomized neural networks. In: Oneto, L., Navarin, N., Sperduti, A., Anguita, D. (eds.) Recent Trends in Learning From Data. SCI, vol. 896, pp. 43–68. Springer, Cham (2020). https://doi.org/10.1007/978-3-030-43883-8_3

13. Gogate, V., Webb, W., Domingos, P.: Learning efficient Markov networks. In: Advances in Neural Information Processing Systems, vol. 23 (2010)

14. Greenewald, K., Zhou, S., Hero, A., III.: Tensor graphical lasso (TeraLasso). J. R. Stat. Soc. Ser. B (Stat. Methodol.) **81**(5), 901–931 (2019)

15. Hallac, D., Park, Y., Boyd, S., Leskovec, J.: Network inference via the time-varying graphical lasso. In: Proceedings of the 23rd ACM SIGKDD International Conference on Knowledge Discovery and Data Mining, pp. 205–213 (2017)

16. Haury, A.C., Mordelet, F., Vera-Licona, P., Vert, J.P.: TIGRESS: trustful inference of gene regulation using stability selection. BMC Syst. Biol. **6**(1), 145 (2012)

17. Heckerman, D., Chickering, D.M., Meek, C., Rounthwaite, R., Kadie, C.: Dependency networks for inference, collaborative filtering, and data visualization. J. Mach. Learn. Res. **1**, 49–75 (2001). https://doi.org/10.1162/153244301753344614

18. Heckerman, D., Geiger, D., Chickering, D.M.: Learning Bayesian networks: the combination of knowledge and statistical data. Mach. Learn. **20**(3), 197–243 (1995)

19. Hsieh, C.J., Sustik, M.A., Dhillon, I.S., Ravikumar, P., et al.: QUIC: quadratic approximation for sparse inverse covariance estimation. J. Mach. Learn. Res. **15**(1), 2911–2947 (2014)

20. Imani, S., Shrivastava, H.: tGLAD: a sparse graph recovery based approach for multivariate time series segmentation. In: 8th Workshop on Advanced Analytics and Learning on Temporal Data (AALTD) at ECML-PKDD (2023). https://doi.org/10.48550/arXiv.2303.11647

21. Koller, D., Friedman, N.: Probabilistic Graphical Models: Principles and Techniques. MIT Press (2009)

22. Lee, S.I., Ganapathi, V., Koller, D.: Efficient structure learning of Markov networks using $l_1$-regularization. In: Advances in Neural Information Processing Systems, vol. 19 (2006)

23. Lou, Y., Caruana, R., Gehrke, J., Hooker, G.: Accurate intelligible models with pairwise interactions. In: Proceedings of the 19th ACM SIGKDD International Conference on Knowledge Discovery and Data Mining, pp. 623–631. ACM (2013)

24. Margolin, A.A., et al.: ARACNE: an algorithm for the reconstruction of gene regulatory networks in a mammalian cellular context. BMC Bioinf. **7**, 1–15 (2006)

25. Moerman, T., et al.: GRNBoost2 and Arboreto: efficient and scalable inference of gene regulatory networks. Bioinformatics **35**(12), 2159–2161 (2019)

26. Pearl, J., Mackenzie, D.: The Book of Why: The New Science of Cause and Effect. Basic Books (2018)

27. Pu, X., Cao, T., Zhang, X., Dong, X., Chen, S.: Learning to learn graph topologies. In: Advances in Neural Information Processing Systems, vol. 34 (2021)

28. Rajbhandari, S., Shrivastava, H., He, Y.: AntMan: sparse low-rank compression to accelerate RNN inference. arXiv preprint arXiv:1910.01740 (2019)

29. Ramanujan, V., Wortsman, M., Kembhavi, A., Farhadi, A., Rastegari, M.: What's hidden in a randomly weighted neural network? In: Proceedings of the IEEE/CVF Conference on Computer Vision and Pattern Recognition, pp. 11893–11902 (2020)

30. Rolfs, B., Rajaratnam, B., Guillot, D., Wong, I., Maleki, A.: Iterative thresholding algorithm for sparse inverse covariance estimation. In: Advances in Neural Information Processing Systems, vol. 25, pp. 1574–1582 (2012)
31. Van de Sande, B., et al.: A scalable scenic workflow for single-cell gene regulatory network analysis. Nat. Protoc. **15**(7), 2247–2276 (2020)
32. Scutari, M.: Learning Bayesian networks with the bnlearn R package. J. Stat. Softw. **35**(3), 1–22 (2010)
33. Shrivastava, H.: On using inductive biases for designing deep learning architectures. Ph.D. thesis, Georgia Institute of Technology (2020)
34. Shrivastava, H., Bart, E., Price, B., Dai, H., Dai, B., Aluru, S.: Cooperative neural networks (CoNN): exploiting prior independence structure for improved classification. arXiv preprint arXiv:1906.00291 (2019)
35. Shrivastava, H., Chajewska, U.: Methods for recovering conditional independence graphs: a survey. arXiv preprint arXiv:2211.06829 (2022)
36. Shrivastava, H., Chajewska, U.: Neural graphical models. In: Proceedings of the 17th European Conference on Symbolic and Quantitative Approaches to Reasoning with Uncertainty (ECSQARU), August 2023. https://doi.org/10.48550/arXiv.2210.00453
37. Shrivastava, H., Chajewska, U., Abraham, R., Chen, X.: A deep learning approach to recover conditional independence graphs. In: NeurIPS 2022 Workshop: New Frontiers in Graph Learning (2022). https://openreview.net/forum?id=kEwzoI3Am4c
38. Shrivastava, H., Chajewska, U., Abraham, R., Chen, X.: uGLAD: sparse graph recovery by optimizing deep unrolled networks. arXiv preprint arXiv:2205.11610 (2022)
39. Shrivastava, H., et al.: GLAD: learning sparse graph recovery. arXiv preprint arXiv:1906.00271 (2019)
40. Shrivastava, H., Garg, A., Cao, Y., Zhang, Y., Sainath, T.: Echo state speech recognition. In: 2021 IEEE International Conference on Acoustics, Speech and Signal Processing (ICASSP), ICASSP 2021, pp. 5669–5673. IEEE (2021)
41. Shrivastava, H., Huddar, V., Bhattacharya, S., Rajan, V.: Classification with imbalance: a similarity-based method for predicting respiratory failure. In: 2015 IEEE International Conference on Bioinformatics and Biomedicine (BIBM), pp. 707–714. IEEE (2015)
42. Shrivastava, H., Huddar, V., Bhattacharya, S., Rajan, V.: System and method for predicting health condition of a patient. US Patent 11,087,879, 10 August 2021
43. Shrivastava, H., Zhang, X., Aluru, S., Song, L.: GRNUlar: gene regulatory network reconstruction using unrolled algorithm from single cell RNA-sequencing data. bioRxiv (2020)
44. Shrivastava, H., Zhang, X., Song, L., Aluru, S.: GRNUlar: a deep learning framework for recovering single-cell gene regulatory networks. J. Comput. Biol. **29**(1), 27–44 (2022)
45. Singh, M., Valtorta, M.: An algorithm for the construction of Bayesian network structures from data. In: Uncertainty in Artificial Intelligence, pp. 259–265. Elsevier (1993)
46. Städler, N., Bühlmann, P.: Missing values: sparse inverse covariance estimation and an extension to sparse regression. Stat. Comput. **22**(1), 219–235 (2012)
47. United States Department of Health and Human Services (US DHHS), Centers of Disease Control and Prevention (CDC), National Center for Health Statistics (NCHS), Division of Vital Statistics (DVS): Birth Cohort Linked Birth - Infant Death Data Files, 2004–2015, compiled from data provided by the 57 vital statistics jurisdictions through the Vital Statistics Cooperative Program, on CDC WONDER On-line Database. https://www.cdc.gov/nchs/data_access/vitalstatsonline.htm

48. Vân Anh Huynh-Thu, A.I., Wehenkel, L., Geurts, P.: Inferring regulatory networks from expression data using tree-based methods. PLoS ONE **5**(9), e12776 (2010)
49. Wang, Y., Jang, B., Hero, A.: The Sylvester Graphical Lasso (SyGlasso). In: International Conference on Artificial Intelligence and Statistics, pp. 1943–1953. PMLR (2020)
50. Williams, D.R.: Beyond Lasso: a survey of nonconvex regularization in Gaussian graphical models (2020)
51. Yu, J., Smith, V.A., Wang, P.P., Hartemink, A.J., Jarvis, E.D.: Using Bayesian network inference algorithms to recover molecular genetic regulatory networks. In: International Conference on Systems Biology, vol. 2002 (2002)
52. Yu, Y., Chen, J., Gao, T., Yu, M.: DAG-GNN: DAG structure learning with graph neural networks. In: International Conference on Machine Learning, pp. 7154–7163. PMLR (2019)
53. Zhang, M., Jiang, S., Cui, Z., Garnett, R., Chen, Y.: D-VAE: a variational autoencoder for directed acyclic graphs. In: Advances in Neural Information Processing Systems, vol. 32 (2019)
54. Zheng, X., Aragam, B., Ravikumar, P.K., Xing, E.P.: DAGs with NO TEARS: Continuous optimization for structure learning. In: Advances in Neural Information Processing Systems, vol. 31, pp. 9472–9483 (2018)
55. Zheng, X., Dan, C., Aragam, B., Ravikumar, P., Xing, E.: Learning sparse nonparametric DAGs. In: International Conference on Artificial Intelligence and Statistics, pp. 3414–3425. PMLR (2020)

# Multi-modal Biomarker Extraction Framework for Therapy Monitoring of Social Anxiety and Depression Using Audio and Video

Tobias Weise[1,2]✉ , Paula Andrea Pérez-Toro[1,3]✉ , Andrea Deitermann[4],
Bettina Hoffmann[4], Kubilay can Demir[2] , Theresa Straetz[4], Elmar Nöth[1] ,
Andreas Maier[1] , Thomas Kallert[4], and Seung Hee Yang[2]

[1] Pattern Recognition Lab, Friedrich-Alexander-Universität Erlangen-Nürnberg,
Erlangen, Germany
{paula.andrea.perez,elmar.noeth,andreas.maier}@fau.de
[2] Speech and Language Processing Lab, Friedrich-Alexander-Universität
Erlangen-Nürnberg, Erlangen, Germany
{tobias.weise,kubilay.c.demir,seung.hee.yang}@fau.de
[3] GITA Lab, Faculty of Engineering, Universidad de Antioquia, Medellín, Colombia
[4] Psychiatric Health Care Facilities of Upper Franconia, Bayreuth, Germany
{andrea.deitermann,bettina.hoffmann,theresa.straetz,
thomas.kallert}@gebo-med.de

**Abstract.** This paper introduces a framework that can be used for
feature extraction, relevant to monitoring the speech therapy progress
of individuals suffering from social anxiety or depression. It operates
multi-modal (decision fusion) by incorporating audio and video recordings of a patient and the corresponding interviewer, at two separate test
assessment sessions. The used data is provided by an ongoing project
in a day-hospital and outpatient setting in Germany, with the goal of
investigating whether an established speech therapy group program for
adolescents, which is implemented in a stationary and semi-stationary
setting, can be successfully carried out via telemedicine. The features
proposed in this multi-modal approach could form the basis for interpretation and analysis by medical experts and therapists, in addition to
acquired data in the form of questionnaires. Extracted audio features
focus on prosody (intonation, stress, rhythm, and timing), as well as
predictions from a deep neural network model, which is inspired by the
Pleasure, Arousal, Dominance (PAD) emotional model space. Video features are based on a pipeline that is designed to enable visualization
of the interaction between the patient and the interviewer in terms of
Facial Emotion Recognition (FER), utilizing the *mini-Xception* network
architecture.

**Keywords:** multi-modal · biomarkers · prosody · emotion
recognition · depression · social anxiety · telemedicine

T. Weise and P. A. Pérez-Toro—Authors contributed equally to this work.

# 1   Introduction

In today's fast-paced and interconnected world, social anxiety and depression have emerged as significant mental health problems, particularly among teenagers. The developmental stage of adolescence, coupled with the complex social dynamics and high expectations, creates a breeding ground for the manifestation of these psychological disorders. Social anxiety, characterized by excessive fear and impaired self-consciousness in social situations, and depression, a pervasive sense of sadness and despair, can severely impair a teenager's emotional well-being, academic performance, and overall quality of life [17].

Recognizing the impact of these mental health conditions, professionals have increasingly turned to therapy as an essential aspect for remedying social anxiety and depression in teenagers. Therapy offers a safe and supportive space where adolescents can openly express their thoughts, feelings, and fears while receiving guidance and evidence-based interventions to promote healing and growth. Through various therapeutic approaches, ranging from cognitive-behavioral therapy to mindfulness-based techniques, these sessions aim to equip teenagers with the necessary tools and coping mechanisms to navigate social challenges, overcome negative thought patterns, and regain control over their lives [20].

A partnering medical institution in Germany performs tele-group therapies, addressing the pragmatic-communicative disorder/uncertainties of participating teenagers [26]. These adolescents are diagnosed (*ICD-11-Code 6A01.22*) with some form of social anxiety, depression, and developmental language disorder with impairment of mainly pragmatic language [32]. The aim of this data collection is to answer the question of whether or not it is possible to provide therapy to patients in a remote setting effectively. Therefore, this current study uses data from three already recorded patients in order to answer the question, which automatically extracted multi-modal biomarkers can be used for analyzing and evaluating the development of patients in such a remote therapy setting. The provided data includes two recordings with the patient and the interviewer at two different points in time: one before the remote therapy started and one after a set amount of such therapy sessions.

Data is in the form of video recordings of the patient, as well as the interviewer, including the accompanying audio tracks. This is done to enable multi-modal approaches toward feature extraction and analysis. In this area two paradigms of fusion are commonly used: *feature fusion* and *decision fusion*. Feature fusion focuses on combining features extracted from different sources or modalities to improve the discriminative power of a classifier. Here, the idea is to encode complementary information from the different sources to create a unified feature representation that captures the most relevant aspects of the data. Typical methods involve early fusion, late fusion, or intermediate fusion, indicating at which point the features from different modalities are combined within the architecture. Decision fusion, on the other hand, combines the decisions or predictions made by multiple classifiers. In doing so, and in contrast to the fusion of features, decision fusion aims at leveraging the diversity and complementary strengths of multiple classifiers to improve the final decision. It can typically involve techniques like majority voting, weighted voting, or rule-based fusion, in order to combine the different classifier outputs.

The effects that the interviewer can have in relation to depressed mood have already been an area of research in the 1970s [6]. Data in the form of a mental health assessment questionnaire was collected from over 1000 individuals from six different interviewers. The authors discovered a significant difference in responses between one interviewer and the other five interviewers when analyzing 15 psycho-social tests. They also offer suggestions in order to minimize the interviewer's effects in such studies. [2] hypothesize that motivational interviewing may have a positive effect on psychotherapy and drug therapy for depression. They argue that the reason for this lies in focusing on two key aspects that are closely associated with depression: boosting intrinsic motivation and addressing ambivalence towards change. Similar efforts have been made by [9] to compare the effect of motivational interviews with conventional care on the depression scale scores of adolescents with obesity/overweight.

For the envisioned system, used for evaluating the progress of remote therapy of adolescents suffering from depression, we investigated different multi-modal biomarkers. These could be used in conjunction with the paradigm of decision fusion in the future, or can already provide a basis for interpretation and analysis by medical experts. A particular focus was put on finding methods that were also able to analyze the interaction between the patient and the interviewer.

## 2   Data

The data used for this work is collected in a project from an in-day hospital and outpatient setting in Germany (GeBO[1]). This project aims to investigate whether their established speech therapy group program for adolescents with social anxiety or depression, which is implemented in a stationary and semi-stationary setting, can be successfully carried out via telemedicine (i.e., remote monitoring). With their teletherapy program, they hope to provide a sense of achievement for teenagers, enabling them to start everyday communication with more confidence. The goal for the participants is to learn to react flexibly in challenging situations and to utilize their own resources.

It is planned to record between 20 to 60 participants during this ongoing study, however, at the current state and for this work, only the recordings of three patients were available: *A0034* (male), *B0072* (female), and *I0038* (female). Participants are aged between 14 and 17 and a psychiatric underlying condition must be diagnosed or there must be a "suspicion of" a psychiatric underlying condition. Adolescents who are undergoing inpatient child and adolescent psychiatric treatment cannot participate.

Therapy is performed in groups of two to three teenagers. Participation takes place from a quiet location using a tablet with a SIM card (which is provided). The program consists of 18 sessions of 60 min each over a period of 6 weeks. A

---

[1] https://www.gebo-med.de/tele-just.

diagnostic session is performed in presence before and after the therapy phase, for this paper these are referenced as T1 (before, no therapy) and T2 (after 18 therapy sessions). These two points of measurement and assessment of therapy effectiveness sessions (i.e., at T1 and T2) involve different questionnaires and three performed exercises called: *Reise*, *ACL*, and *NuS*. Here, the latter is a read speech test, where the teenagers have to read the "Northwind and the Sun" text. The other two include spontaneous speech between the patient and the interviewer, where one involves describing a place where they would like to travel to (*Reise*), and the other involves performing and discussing a certain task (*ACL*).

Recordings and thus the provided data were performed by the therapists via Open Broadcaster Software (OBS). It shows the larger video of the patient (camera setup) and the smaller video of the interviewer (laptop webcam). In total, six such OBS recordings are provided per patient: exercises *NuS*, *ACL*, and *Reise* at T1 and T2. An example of this is shown in Figs. 1 and 3. Both the teenager and the interviewer wear a headset for recording the matching audio into separate channels with ideally only one voice per channel.

## 3  Audio Biomarkers

This section focuses on the audio features that were extracted from the individual OBS recordings, which can then be compared and analyzed for T1 and T2, in order to see potential changes in the patient's behavior related to speech. An overview of the extraction pipeline can be seen in Fig. 1. First, *ffmpeg* is used to extract $(160kb/s, 16kHz)$ the two audio channels as single wav-files, one containing the interviewer's speech and the other containing the patients' speech, from the OBS recorded video.

No further pre-processing (e.g. any form of signal normalization) is done after the audio channel extraction. The reason for this is not to falsify the information content contained within the recordings. For example, the average energy contour is used as an extracted biomarker, which would be distorted if energy normalization (over the entire recording) was performed beforehand.

Furthermore, it should be noted that if there is no strict audio channel separation between the patient and the interviewer (at the time of recording), some additional pre-processing might be necessary. This could involve techniques like voice activity detection (VAD) or speaker diarisation.

The following subsections show specifically what audio-based features were extracted, and Fig. 1 shows what input was used for each.

### 3.1  Prosody

We chose to extract and analyze prosody-based features, which refer to rhythm, intonation, and stress patterns in speech since they can be impacted by social anxiety and depression [7]. We split these prosodic features into two groups, where we combine rhythm (3.1), intonation and stress (3.1).

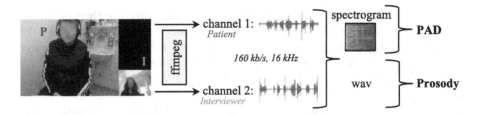

**Fig. 1.** Audio-based emotion biomarker extraction pipeline.

Prosodic features can be affected by social anxiety since individuals suffering from it may exhibit certain speech patterns, including a tendency to speak softly or rapidly, with increased pitch variability or reduced vocal modulation. These prosodic alterations may result from heightened self-consciousness, fear of judgment, or a desire to avoid drawing attention. Such atypical prosody can impact social interactions by influencing how others perceive the person's speech, potentially leading to social difficulties.

When dealing with depression, which is a mood disorder characterized by persistent sadness, loss of interest or pleasure, and other symptoms, prosodic features can be affected as a result of the emotional and cognitive changes associated with this condition. Patients suffering from this may exhibit flatter or monotonous speech, reduced speech rate, and decreased vocal energy [14, 22, 25]. These alterations in prosody can reflect the overall emotional state and can contribute to communication difficulties.

It's important to note that prosodic changes can occur in various speech disorders and conditions, so they are not exclusive to social anxiety and depression. However, recognizing and understanding these prosodic alterations can be valuable for clinicians, as they may provide insights into a person's emotional well-being and aid in diagnosing or monitoring these conditions.

**Intonation and Stress.** For prosodic features that are related to intonation and stress, we chose to extract and analyze the following: fundamental frequency (F0) contour (based on 40 ms chunks), and energy contour (computed over the voiced and unvoiced segments). In contrast and naturally, only voiced segments were used for the F0 contour. Based on these contours, mean and standard deviation functionals were computed.

**Rhythm and Timing.** We also chose to extract prosodic features that can be broadly regarded as duration, and more precisely rhythm and timing based. Here, from the speech and pause duration we extracted the mean, standard deviation, minimum and maximum values, as well as the voiced rate (VRT). The latter is also known as speech rate and it expresses the speed at which a person speaks.

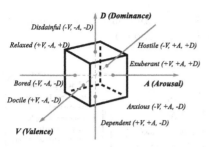

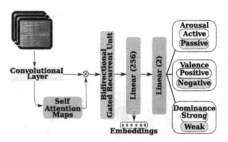

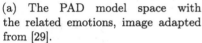

(a) The PAD model space with the related emotions, image adapted from [29].

(b) Architecture of three pre-trained models and PAD-based models, taken from [21].

**Fig. 2.** Pleasure, Arousal, and Dominance (PAD) emotional model-related information, which is part of the audio-based extracted features used in the proposed framework. Note: "Pleasure" was replaced with "Valence" for this work.

## 3.2 PAD Model

The Pleasure, Arousal, and Dominance [18] emotional model (PAD) represents and quantifies emotions in a three-dimensional space, where the dimensions relate to pleasant-unpleasant (pleasure), calm-agitated (arousal), or dominant-submissive (dominance). Figure 2a shows this space, however, for this work, we changed the name of the pleasure dimension to valence.

We follow the same approach as [21] and train in total three models using the Interactive Emotional Dyadic Motion Capture (IEMOCAP) database [5]. It should be noted that this database contains only English speech, which might have an impact on the results, however, there is no alternative/equivalent German database available. The three models can perform binary classification between active vs. passive arousal (accuracy = 67%), positive vs. negative valence (accuracy = 88%), and strong vs. weak dominance (accuracy = 80%).

Compared to the individual and classical prosodic features, such a model can be seen more as a holistic approach toward emotion recognition based on acoustic clues. The idea is to use the outputs of the three models in order to place the speech patterns of a patient inside this three-dimensional space at T1 and, then again, at T2 in order to compare some differences caused by the therapy sessions [19].

The architecture of the PAD model(s) can be seen in Fig. 2b. As input, it takes three log magnitude Mel spectrograms, computed with different time resolutions of 16, 25, and 45 ms and a sequence length of 500 ms. A convolutional layer extracts spacial information within the spectrum(s), while self-attention, as well as bidirectional Gated Recurrent Units (GRU), encode context across the convolved sequence of spectrograms. This is followed by a linear layer with 256 units and dropout regularization ($p = 0.3$), and a final linear layer with 2 units in order to obtain the posterior probabilities, using a Sigmoid activation function.

This activation was considered to observe the contribution of each dimension (e.g. active vs. passive arousal) by taking independent outputs.

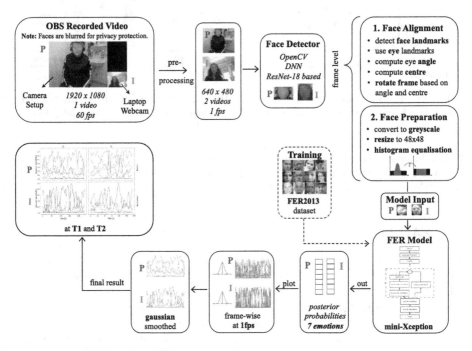

**Fig. 3.** Video-based emotion biomarker extraction pipeline centered around a deep FER-model. (mini-Xception figure taken from [3])

## 4   Video Biomarkers

This section focuses on the video features that were extracted from the individual OBS recordings, which can then be compared and analyzed for T1 and T2, in order to see potential changes in the patient's behavior concerning facial expressions [8]. Here, we focus on proposing a method that can be used to analyze the interaction between the patient and the interviewer. This is possible since the OBS recording includes both of these recordings (Fig. 3).

Facial emotions can have a significant impact on patients with depression [4,11,15,23] and social anxiety [30,31]. In both conditions, facial emotions can influence the individual's perception of themselves and others. Negative facial expressions of a conversation partner may reinforce negative self-perceptions, exacerbate symptoms, and contribute to a cycle of negative thoughts and emotions. However, it is important to note that the impact that facial emotions have varies among individuals. Furthermore, patients with depression often struggle with anhedonia, which is the inability to experience pleasure (valence in this paper) or derive enjoyment from activities that would typically be enjoyable. This reduced ability to experience positive emotions can make it challenging for them to reflect or genuinely respond to happy facial expressions (e.g. from an interviewer). Even if they intellectually understand that the other person is expressing happiness, they may have difficulty emotionally connecting or reciprocating those positive emotions [13,24]. A similar effect can occur in the case of social anxiety, where individuals may also struggle to reflect happy facial emotions due to their preoccupation with their own perceived flaws, social performance, or potential negative judgments from others, making it challenging for them to authentically reflect positive emotions. Additionally, patients suffering from social anxiety may have difficulties with emotional regulation. Their anxiety may cause emotional states such as tension, fear, or worry to override positive emotions. Consequently, even if they recognize a happy facial expression, their internal emotional state may hinder their ability to reflect or reciprocate those emotions effectively [16,27].

The proposed method of extracting facial emotions from the patients, as well as the interviewer's face, is intended to shed light on the above-mentioned phenomena(s). Ideally, changes in the isolated behavior of the patient, as well as in the interaction with the interviewer can be made visible, when comparing T1 and T2 and thus providing an effective monitoring of the therapy progress of the individual patient.

### 4.1   Face Emotion Recognition

This subsection goes into more detail on how the facial emotion recognition (FER) system functions, with a schematic overview in Fig. 3. The entire pipeline is implemented using Python. Starting point is an OBS recording of a therapy assessment session (at T1 or T2), showing both the patient and the interviewer, (for this work) recorded at 1920 × 1080 at 60 frames per second (fps). For this part of the feature extraction, the audio portion of the recordings is discarded, and only video information is further processed. This initial recording is split into two separate videos, which are scaled to be of the same size 640 × 480, and down-sampled to 1 fps. Whilst it is possible to implement this pipeline using a higher frame rate, we argue that 1 fps is sufficient, considering that the therapy assessment sessions can take up to 20 min of time. The next step is to apply a face detector to the, now two separate, videos. For this work, we used the *OpenCV* toolkit (wrapper package for Python bindings), which provides a deep neural network (DNN) based face detector, utilizing the *Resnet-18* architecture [12]. After this frame-level detection of faces, they need to be aligned before further processing. This is done based on facial landmark detection (*OpenCV*), where only the landmarks of both eyes are used and averaged to one point per eye. This enables the computation of the angle between the line connecting the two average eye points. Next, the entire frame is rotated using a 2-dimensional rotation matrix, which is based on the angle and the determined rotation center of the current frame. As a last step before model input, the frame is converted to greyscale, resized to 48 × 48, and histogram equalization is performed.

This pre-processing is necessary because the used deep neural network is trained with the FER2013 dataset [10]. It was introduced at the International Conference on Machine Learning (ICML) in 2013, where each face has been labeled based on seven different emotional classes (*angy, disgust, fear, happy, sad, surprise, neutral*). Furthermore, the images contained in this database are in greyscale, measuring 48 × 48 pixels.

The deep architecture used in this pipeline is called *mini-Xception* [3], which was introduced in 2017, is designed to perform image classification tasks, and has proven especially effective in tasks such as object recognition. The core idea behind Xception is the concept of *depthwise separable convolutions*, splitting the traditional spatial and channel-wise convolution operation into two separate layers, which enables more parameter-efficient computation. The Xception architecture stacks such separated convolutions to form an exceptionally deep structure, hence the name "Xception", which stands for "extreme inception". This also implies that it utilizes a modified Inception [28] module, where the traditional 3 × 3 convolutions are replaced with depthwise separable convolutions.

After the individual and pre-processed faces are input into the model, the output is the posterior probabilities of the seven different emotional categories for the given face image. This is performed for both pre-processed videos (patient and interviewer, based on the original unified OBS recording) at the frame level with 1 fps. Consequently, enabling the visualization of these predicted face emotion posterior probabilities over the duration of a therapy assessment session (T1/T2), with a "prediction rate" of 1 Hz. In order to make these plots more interpretable, a 1-dimensional Gaussian smoothing is applied, where the width parameter is proportional to the overall duration of the individual assessment session. Refer to Sect. 5.2 for more details on the resulting final plot.

## 5    Results

The data collection process of the study mentioned in Sect. 2 is still ongoing. For this reason, we only have recordings of three patients at the moment of writing this paper. From this data, we show results of the proposed multi-modal feature extraction of all patients, performing the same exercise out of the three in total performed exercises, which is *Reise*. The remainder of this section is split into results from the extracted audio and video features.

### 5.1    Audio Biomarkers

Results from the extracted audio biomarkers are displayed in a tabular format. Table 1 shows the prosody-based features that are related to intonation and stress in the form of mean and standard deviation of the F0 and energy contours. Table 2 also shows prosody-related results, related to the rhythm and timing of the patient and the interviewer at T1 and T2. Extracted PAD results, meaning the functionals of the outputs from the three trained models, are shown in Table 3. In detail, displayed values are the mean and standard deviation of

**Table 1.** Prosody (intonation and stress): mean and standard deviation for F0 and energy contour.

| Func. | T1 | | T2 | |
|---|---|---|---|---|
| | Patient | Inter. | Patient | Inter. |
| F0 | 124.00 | 206.85 | 121.97 | 211.50 |
| Contour | ±41.10 | ±53.65 | ±45.05 | ±54.42 |
| Energy | 3.6e−5 | 4.5e−5 | 5.7e−6 | 1.1e−5 |
| Contour | ±9.4e−5 | ±1.7e−4 | ±2.8e−5 | ±9.4e−5 |

(a) Intonation and stress related values of patient *A0034*.

| Func. | T1 | | T2 | |
|---|---|---|---|---|
| | Patient | Inter. | Patient | Inter. |
| F0 | 222.29 | 239.74 | 233.26 | 219.29 |
| Contour | ±30.10 | ±66.67 | ±39.35 | ±68.73 |
| Energy | 2.9e−5 | 2.9e−6 | 4.8e−5 | 7.4e−6 |
| Contour | ±1.16e−4 | ±1.9e−6 | ±1.2e−4 | ±5.5e−5 |

(b) Intonation and stress related values of patient *B0072*.

| Func. | T1 | | T2 | |
|---|---|---|---|---|
| | Patient | Inter. | Patient | Inter. |
| F0 | 220.17 | 232.80 | 231.56 | 237.74 |
| Contour | ±43.93 | ±63.94 | ±31.89 | ±75.82 |
| Energy | 1.4e−5 | 6.3e−6 | 3.6e−5 | 8.1e−6 |
| Contour | ±7.3e−5 | ±3.7e−5 | ±1.1e−4 | ±1.2e−4 |

(c) Intonation and stress related values of patient *I0038*.

the specific model (e.g. Valence), across the entire exercise. As the predicted output of such a model is complementary, we show the higher of the two values (in regards to the patient) for T1 and T2. The used acronyms are based on the PAD model(s), with "AA" and "PA" standing for Active and Passive Arousal, "PV" and "NV" for Positive and Negative Valence, and "SD" and "WD" are short for Strong and Weak Dominance.

## 5.2   Video Biomarkers

The chosen type of visualization for the extracted FER-based video biomarkers is the final figure in the bottom left of the schematic overview in Fig. 3. This plot is created for each patient, and for each of the three exercises that are performed by the individual at the two therapy assessment sessions (T1 and T2). In this work, we show results based on one of these three exercises, called *Reise*, in Figs. 4a, 4b, and 4c. These plots show the posterior probabilities of the FER model, with a prediction output frequency of 1hz. Each of the seven different predicted emotions is displayed as a separate color. The vertical plane shares the

**Table 2.** Prosody (rhythm and timing): mean and standard deviation, min- and maximum speech and pause duration, and voiced rate (VRT).

| Func. | T1 | | T2 | |
|---|---|---|---|---|
| | Patient | Inter. | Patient | Inter. |
| Speech Duration | 11.90 ±10.16 | 10.44 ±13.37 | 7.00 ±6.31 | 10.47 ±8.90 |
| Pause Duration | 4.60 ±5.74 | 4.35 ±3.60 | 3.85 ±3.15 | 4.51 ±4.82 |
| VRT | 1.43 | 1.50 | 0.77 | 1.02 |
| min/max Speech | 1.31/37.40 | 0.35/52.37 | 0.20/20.40 | 0.19/24.02 |
| min/max Pause | 0.67/22.79 | 0.78/13.09 | 0.70/10.40 | 0.66/14.63 |

(a) Rhythm and timing related values of patient *A0034*.

| Func. | T1 | | T2 | |
|---|---|---|---|---|
| | Patient | Inter. | Patient | Inter. |
| Speech Duration | 11.65 ±17.26 | 7.75 ±7.59 | 15.81 ±28.23 | 5.62 ±5.54 |
| Pause Duration | 4.51 ±4.88 | 3.30 ±2.80 | 4.68 ±3.42 | 2.35 ±1.16 |
| VRT | 1.24 | 0.68 | 1.79 | 0.73 |
| min/max Speech | 0.41/48.71 | 1.38/19.87 | 0.54/72.27 | 1.06/21.61 |
| min/max Pause | 0.58/14.71 | 0.07/9.89 | 1.50/9.89 | 1.03/4.87 |

(b) Rhythm and timing related values of patient *B0072*.

| Func. | T1 | | T2 | |
|---|---|---|---|---|
| | Patient | Inter. | Patient | Inter. |
| Speech Duration | 7.11 ±10.18 | 13.69 ±16.45 | 6.03 ±10.87 | 7.42 ±8.15 |
| Pause Duration | 3.17 ±3.21 | 4.60 ±2.63 | 2.56 ±1.57 | 3.46 ±3.30 |
| VRT | 0.89 | 1.33 | 1.14 | 0.58 |
| min/max Speech | 0.73/38.22 | 0.37/42.44 | 0.06/39.59 | 0.17/26.37 |
| min/max Pause | 0.34/10.00 | 0.44/7.73 | 0.73/5.90 | 0.28/11.10 |

(c) Rhythm and timing related values of patient *I0038*.

same time axis since it is based on the video of the patient and the interviewer at that specific assessment session T1. It can therefore be used to analyze the facial emotional actions and reactions between the patient and the interviewer. The plots show both assessments in the form of T1 and T2 (reminder: 18 therapy sessions between them), which in turn enables monitoring of potential changes in the facial emotional reactions of the patient, to those of the interviewer.

**Table 3.** PAD model: mean and standard deviation of the three PAD model outputs. The higher of the two complementary output values (of the patient) is displayed for each of the three models. For an explanation of the acronyms, refer to Figs. 2a and 2b.

| T1 | | | T2 | | |
|---|---|---|---|---|---|
| PAD | Patient | Inter. | PAD | Patient | Inter. |
| NV | 0.63 | 0.55 | NV | 0.59 | 0.32 |
| (V-) | ±0.09 | ±0.24 | (V-) | ±0.07 | ±0.27 |
| AA | 0.82 | 0.70 | AA | 0.91 | 0.70 |
| (A+) | ±0.27 | ±0.30 | (A+) | ±0.16 | ±0.18 |
| SD | 0.55 | 0.43 | WD | 0.53 | 0.33 |
| (D+) | ±0.17 | ±0.22 | (D-) | ±0.16 | ±0.20 |

(a) Patient *A0034*. In this case, the patient shifted from *Hostile (V-, A+, D+)* at T1 to *Anxious (V-, A+, D-)* at T2.

| T1 | | | T2 | | |
|---|---|---|---|---|---|
| PAD | Patient | Inter. | PAD | Patient | Inter. |
| PV | 0.69 | 0.66 | PV | 0.55 | 0.57 |
| (V+) | ±0.35 | ±0.23 | (V+) | ±0.31 | ±0.22 |
| AA | 0.79 | 0.75 | AA | 0.79 | 0.76 |
| (A+) | ±0.18 | ±0.14 | (A+) | ±0.24 | ±0.22 |
| WD | 0.60 | 0.70 | SD | 0.51 | 0.34 |
| (D-) | ±0.28 | ±0.17 | (D+) | ±0.26 | ±0.17 |

(b) Patient *B0072*. In this case, the patient shifted from *Dependent (V+, A+, D-)* at T1 to *Exuberant (V+, A+, D+)* at T2.

| T1 | | | T2 | | |
|---|---|---|---|---|---|
| PAD | Patient | Inter. | PAD | Patient | Inter. |
| PV | 0.60 | 0.61 | NV | 0.66 | 0.74 |
| (V+) | ±0.15 | ±0.27 | (V-) | ±0.09 | ±0.23 |
| AA | 0.85 | 0.72 | AA | 0.86 | 0.74 |
| (A+) | ±0.14 | ±0.19 | (A+) | ±0.25 | ±0.15 |
| WD | 0.58 | 0.64 | SD | 0.54 | 0.30 |
| (D-) | ±0.19 | ±0.18 | (D+) | ±0.18 | ±0.16 |

(c) Patient *I0038*. In this case, the patient shifted from *Dependent (V+, A+, D-)* at T1 to *Hostile (V-, A+, D+)* at T2.

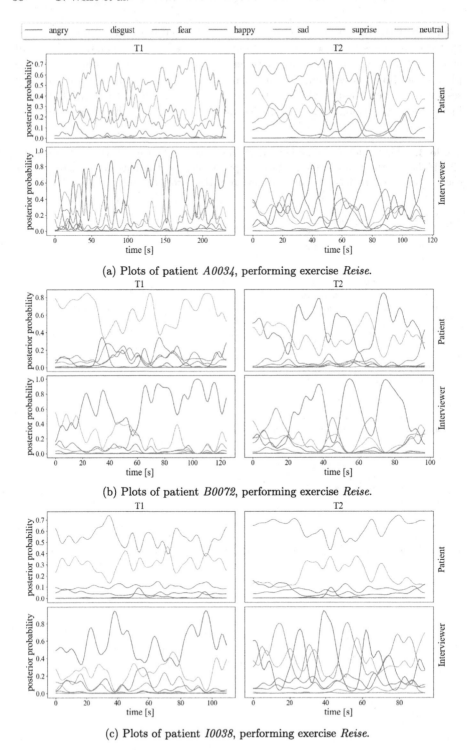

(a) Plots of patient *A0034*, performing exercise *Reise*.

(b) Plots of patient *B0072*, performing exercise *Reise*.

(c) Plots of patient *I0038*, performing exercise *Reise*.

**Fig. 4.** FER posterior probability plots (see Fig. 3) at T1 and T2 for three patients and individual interviewers, highlighting the interaction between them.

# 6   Discussion

The extracted biomarkers in this work are intended to form a basis, in addition to questionnaires that are gathered at the two assessments T1 and T2. It facilitates and supports the interpretation and analysis provided by medical experts and therapists to monitor the progress of the therapy effectively. For the specific project that provided the data used in this work, the motivation is to find out if a remote speech and language therapy setting can be effectively used to treat patients that suffer from social anxiety and depression. At this point, it should also be noted that since this is an ongoing data collection project, there is no "ground truth" in terms of (human) medical experts yet, for the three patients covered in this work. The remainder of this section highlights some potential and preliminary observations on a per-patient basis for each of the three patients.

For patient *A0034* (male), the results of the video biomarkers (see Fig. 4a) suggest an effect that the (remote) therapy of this patient had on his ability to reflect the "Happy" emotion of the interviewer. Another noteworthy observation is the fact that at T2, the FER model detected the "Angry" emotion in the interviewer with around 60% probability. Anger is typically associated with facial expressions involving frowning, tightened eyebrows, and tense facial muscles. On the other hand, when individuals are deep in thought or fully engaged in concentration, they may also display similar facial features. Interesting to note here, and likely not noticed by the interviewer at that time, is that this corresponds to a FER-detected "Fear" spike in the patient. In terms of audio biomarkers, the PAD model (Table 3a) shifted him from "Hostile" at T1, to "Anxious" at T2, caused by a shift from "Weak Dominance" to "Strong Dominance". Interestingly, and in contrast to the patient *I0038*, this did not occur in parallel with an average energy contour increase (Table 1a), but rather a decrease, indicating that more subtle factors impact the "Dominance"-PAD model's predictions. A possible multi-layered cause for this could be the slight drop in F0, the almost halving of the VRT, or the related fact that his pauses became shorter (Table 2a).

When looking at the results of the patient *B0072* (female), in terms of video (Fig. 4b) and audio biomarkers, it is noticeable that the "Exuberant" combined PAD model prediction (Table 3b) correlates with the FER visualization. The results also suggest, that this individual is not only considerably less "Sad", but also more "Happy" at T2 compared to T1, which could be an indicator for successful therapy. Furthermore, to point out some more differences, the average F0 decreased, energy levels increased, and "Weak Dominance" shifted to "Strong Dominance". Overall, of the three patients covered in this work, this patient seems to have improved the most. Regarding pauses and speech content, the interviewer seemed to reduce interaction when the patient spoke more. Furthermore, although the patient had a lower average F0, the interviewer demonstrated an increase in F0, which was consistent across all three cases.

Lastly, results of the patient *I0038* (female), in terms of video biomarkers (Fig. 4c), make it seem evident that the patient's facial emotions did not change from T1 to T2. However, some changes can be observed with regard to audio biomarkers. In terms of PAD models (Table 3c), the mood shifted from

"Dependent" to "Hostile", caused by the change from "Weak Dominance" to "Strong Dominance" and "Positive Valence" to "Negative Valence". The shift in dominance (holistic prediction) is likely connected to the increase in average energy contour, which more than doubled from T1 to T2. Additionally, the maximum pause duration was halved (Table 1c), which could indicate that the individual had less fear of judgment, and did not mentally weigh each answer before speaking.

## 7 Conclusion

We introduced a framework to monitor the progress in the communicative abilities of patients suffering from social anxiety and depression. Using the preliminary data of an ongoing data collection project in this domain, we established a video-based pipeline for FER, which enables tracking of the facial emotional response of a patient and their interviewer. Additionally, we extracted audio-based features that are related to emotional clues, like prosody and functionals of a neural network version of the PAD emotional model as a more holistic approach towards speech emotion recognition. Results show promising trends, that confirm medical assumptions about the potential improvements that individuals, suffering from these conditions, are expected to experience.

This framework can still be expanded upon in future work. For example, it would also be possible to extract certain linguistic features based on an automatic speech recognition (ASR) output. Furthermore, feature fusion between the audio and video modalities could also be investigated, for example utilizing Gated Multimodal Units (GMU) [1]. Related to this, additional speech-based emotion detection algorithms (like the PAD model used in this work) could be explored, to see which results in the best performance.

## References

1. Arevalo, J., Solorio, T., et al.: Gated multimodal units for information fusion. arXiv preprint arXiv:1702.01992 (2017)
2. Arkowitz, H., Burke, B.L.: Motivational interviewing as an integrative framework for the treatment of depression. In: Motivational Interviewing in the Treatment of Psychological Problems, pp. 145–172 (2008)
3. Arriaga, O., Valdenegro-Toro, M., Plöger, P.: Real-time convolutional neural networks for emotion and gender classification. arXiv preprint arXiv:1710.07557 (2017)
4. Bourke, C., Douglas, K., Porter, R.: Processing of facial emotion expression in major depression: a review. Aust. NZ J. Psychiatry 44(8), 681–696 (2010)
5. Busso, C., et al.: IEMOCAP: interactive emotional dyadic motion capture database. Lang. Resour. Eval. 42, 335–359 (2008)
6. Choi, I.C., Comstock, G.W.: Interviewer effect on responses to a questionnaire relating to mood. Am. J. Epidemiol. 101(1), 84–92 (1975)
7. Cummins, N., et al.: A review of depression and suicide risk assessment using speech analysis. Speech Commun. 71, 10–49 (2015)

8. Ekman, P.: Facial expression and emotion. Am. Psychol. **48**(4), 384 (1993)
9. Freira, S., Lemos, M.S.O.: Effect of motivational interviewing on depression scale scores of adolescents with obesity and overweight. Psychiatry Res. **252**, 340–345 (2017)
10. Goodfellow, I.J., et al.: Challenges in representation learning: a report on three machine learning contests. In: Lee, M., Hirose, A., Hou, Z.-G., Kil, R.M. (eds.) ICONIP 2013. LNCS, vol. 8228, pp. 117–124. Springer, Heidelberg (2013). https://doi.org/10.1007/978-3-642-42051-1_16
11. Gur, R.C., Erwin, R.J., et al.: Facial emotion discrimination: Ii. behavioral findings in depression. Psychiatry Res. **42**(3), 241–251 (1992)
12. He, K., Zhang, X., Ren, S., Sun, J.: Deep residual learning for image recognition. In: Proceedings of the IEEE Conference on Computer Vision and Pattern Recognition, pp. 770–778 (2016)
13. Joormann, J., Gotlib, I.H.: Is this happiness I see? Biases in the identification of emotional facial expressions in depression and social phobia. J. Abnorm. Psychol. **115**(4), 705 (2006)
14. Klaar, L., Nagels, A., et al.: Sprachliche besonderheiten in der spontansprache von patientinnen mit depression. Logos (2020)
15. Kohler, C.G., Hoffman, L.J., Eastman, L.B., Healey, K., Moberg, P.J.: Facial emotion perception in depression and bipolar disorder: a quantitative review. Psychiatry Res. **188**(3), 303–309 (2011)
16. Leppänen, J.M., et al.: Depression biases the recognition of emotionally neutral faces. Psychiatry Res. **128**(2), 123–133 (2004)
17. Martin, G.: Depression in teenagers. Curr. Therapeutics **37**(6), 57–67 (1996)
18. Mehrabian, A.: Pleasure-arousal-dominance: a general framework for describing and measuring individual differences in temperament. Curr. Psychol. **14**, 261–292 (1996)
19. Mehrabian, A.: Comparison of the pad and panas as models for describing emotions and for differentiating anxiety from depression. J. Psychopathol. Behav. Assess. **19**, 331–357 (1997)
20. Orsolini, L., Pompili, S., et al.: A systematic review on telemental health in youth mental health: Focus on anxiety, depression and obsessive-compulsive disorder. Medicina **57**(8), 793 (2021)
21. Pérez-Toro, P.A., Bayerl, S.P., et al.: Influence of the interviewer on the automatic assessment of Alzheimer's disease in the context of the Adresso challenge. In: Interspeech, pp. 3785–3789 (2021)
22. Rude, S., Gortner, E.M., Pennebaker, J.: Language use of depressed and depression-vulnerable college students. Cogn. Emotion **18**(8), 1121–1133 (2004)
23. Rutter, L.A., Passell, E., et al.: Depression severity is associated with impaired facial emotion processing in a large international sample. J. Affect. Disord. **275**, 175–179 (2020)
24. Schwartz, G.E., et al.: Facial muscle patterning to affective imagery in depressed and nondepressed subjects. Science **192**(4238), 489–491 (1976)
25. Shugaley, A., Altmann, U., et al.: Klang der depression. Psychotherapeut **67**(2), 158–165 (2022)
26. Strätz, T.: Sprachtherapie mit ängstlichen und depressiven jugendlichen-ein erfahrungsbericht (2022)
27. Surguladze, S., et al.: A differential pattern of neural response toward sad versus happy facial expressions in major depressive disorder. Biol. Psychiat. **57**(3), 201–209 (2005)

28. Szegedy, C., Ioffe, S.o.: Inception-v4, inception-resnet and the impact of residual connections on learning. In: Proceedings of the AAAI Conference on Artificial Intelligence, vol. 31 (2017)
29. Tarasenko, S.: Emotionally colorful reflexive games. arXiv preprint arXiv:1101.0820 (2010)
30. Torro-Alves, N., et al.: Facial emotion recognition in social anxiety: the influence of dynamic information. Psychol. Neurosci. 9(1), 1 (2016)
31. Zhang, Q., Ran, G., Li, X.: The perception of facial emotional change in social anxiety: an ERP study. Front. Psychol. 9, 1737 (2018)
32. Zwirnmann, S., et al.: Fachbeitrag: Sprachliche und emotional-soziale beeinträchtigungen. komorbiditäten und wechselwirkungen. Vierteljahresschrift für Heilpädagogik und ihre Nachbargebiete (2023)

# RobustSsF: Robust Missing Modality Brain Tumor Segmentation with Self-supervised Learning-Based Scenario-Specific Fusion

Jeongwon Lee[✉] and Dae-Shik Kim

KAIST, 291 Daehak-Ro, Yuseong-Gu, Daejeon 34141, South Korea
{gardenlee21,daeshik}@kaist.ac.kr

**Abstract.** All modalities of Magnetic Resonance Imaging (MRI) have an essential role in diagnosing brain tumors, but there are some challenges posed by missing or incomplete modalities in multimodal MRI. Existing models have failed to achieve robust performance across all scenarios. To address this issue, this paper proposes a novel 4encoder-4decoder architecture that incorporates both "dedicated" and "single" models. Our model includes multiple Scenario-specific Fusion (SsF) decoders that construct different features depending on the missing modality scenarios. To train our model, we introduce a novel self-supervised learning-based loss function called Couple Regularization (CReg) to achieve robust learning and the Lifelong Learning Strategy (LLS) to enhance model performance. The experimental results on BraTS2018 demonstrate that RobustSsF has successfully improved robustness by reducing standard deviations from 12 times to 76 times lower, also achieving state-of-the-art results in all scenarios when the T1ce modality is missing.

**Keywords:** Missing modality brain tumor segmentation · Robustness · Regularization

## 1 Introduction

Magnetic Resonance Imaging (MRI) is crucial for brain tumor diagnosis due to its excellent spatial resolution. Different MRI images such as FLAIR, T1, T2, and T1ce are collected to identify key tumor regions for diagnosis. Each key tumor region is segmented based on different modalities [10]. However, situations may arise where one or more modalities cannot be collected, hampering the performance of brain tumor segmentation and diagnosis. This situation is known as missing-modality, and it has been a challenging topic of research for deep learning and medical imaging practitioners over the last decade [1,18]. Developing flexible models that can operate when one or more modalities are missing has been the focus of intense research.

© The Author(s), under exclusive license to Springer Nature Switzerland AG 2024
A. K. Maier et al. (Eds.): ML4MHD 2023, LNCS 14315, pp. 43–53, 2024.
https://doi.org/10.1007/978-3-031-47679-2_4

Based on the aforementioned four modalities, there are a total of 15 multi-modal combinations, also called scenarios, depending on the presence or absence of each modality. There is a full-modality scenario and 14 missing-modality scenarios. In the research community, missing-modality models for brain tumor segmentation are broadly classified into "dedicated" and "single" models, based on how they deal with scenarios. "Dedicated" models train individual models for each scenario, such as [2,7,8,14] models are co-trained with full-modality and [2,14] proposed structures that co-train full-modality and missing-modality paths. Developing different models for each scenario could be both time-consuming and computationally challenging. In contrast, "single" models train one model for all scenarios, making it scenario-invariant and more favorable for clinical applications. Some examples include [3,5,6,16,17]. Since one model covers all scenarios, "single" models is more suitable for clinical application than "dedicated" models.

However, there is still a severe problem that all models have not been solved. The problem is that the model's performance varies significantly depending on which modality is missing. As can be seen in Table 1 (3.2 Results and Analysis), severe performance degradation is observed when the T1ce modality is missing in "dedicated" and "single" models both. T1ce modality can only be scanned after injection of the contrast agent unlike the other three modalities, making it challenging to collect. Also, it contains crucial information for all segmentation labels. This indicated that the model's robustness is low, making it difficult to apply in clinical settings.

To tackle this, this paper proposes a new structure and learning process specialized for all missing-modality scenarios that are different from the brain tumor segmentation model in a full-modality scenario. First, we designed a novel 4encoder-4decoder architecture by adding the elements of the "dedicated" model to the "single" model. Unlike the previous "single" models that deal with all modality scenarios with only one model, the proposed model is a new structure that incorporates the structure of a dedicated model by expanding a fusion decoder with one full-modality decoder and two missing-modality decoders. These are Scenario-specific Fusion (SsF) decoders that receive different features depending on which modality is missing. Second, a novel self-supervised learning-based loss function is proposed for improving the robustness of the model in all scenarios by utilizing the new self-evident fact that has not been used, which is specific to the missing modality brain tumor segmentation field. We named our new loss function Couple Regularization (CReg). Additionally, Lifelong Learning Strategy (LLS) was also employed to achieve a more comprehensive performance. Lifelong learning is a field that aims to enable machine learning models to continuously learn and adapt to new information throughout their lifespan [9,12,13,15]. This is distinct from traditional machine learning, where models are trained on a fixed dataset and applied to new data without further adjustment.

Experimental results indicate that our proposed model has successfully enhanced the robustness compared to other state-of-the-art models, by exhibiting more than a 20-fold reduction in the standard deviation, which represents the performance gap across all scenarios. Specifically, we achieved not only state-of-the-art results in TC and ET labels for all scenarios, where T1ce was missing but also in all other challenging scenarios and labels.

## 2   Method

### 2.1   Overall Architecture

The proposed model consists of a 4-encoder-4-decoder architecture. All four encoders are modality-specific encoders that use the 3D U-Net encoder [4], similar to other missing modality brain tumor segmentation models with encoder-decoder structures [5,16,17]. To preserve the information of each modality as much as possible, a different encoder is used for each modality. Although the structure of all encoders is the same, the weights are not shared and are trained separately. Each encoder generates four feature maps - one feature map for each stage, as shown in Fig. 1.

$$[F_{m_1}, F_{m_2}, F_{m_3}, F_{m_4}] = \mathbf{E}_m(I_m), \tag{1}$$

where the number for stages is 4, $\mathbf{E}_m$ is each modality-specific encoder for the modality $m \in \{$FLAIR, T1c, T1, T2$\}$, $I_m \in R^{W \times H \times Z}$ means each modality image, the size of feature maps are $F_{m_s} \in R^{\frac{W}{2^s} \times \frac{H}{2^s} \times \frac{Z}{2^s}}$ for each $s \in [1, 2, 3, 4]$.

The decoder we propose is divided into two main parts. The first part consists of three scenario-specific decoders specialized in fusion for the missing modality scenarios. The explanation of the first part will be given in the following section. The second part is a single modality-invariant decoder with the U-Net decoder structure. The modality-invariant decoder extracts the feature maps from each modality-specific encoder and uses them to segment each modality image separately. That is, the feature maps of each modality are passed through a single modality-invariant decoder that shares weights to predict the segmentation map in each modality. It helps the scenario-specific decoders to equally learn all information about modalities.

### 2.2   Self-supervised Learning-Based Scenario-Specific Fusion

A "single" model for missing modality brain tumor segmentation aims to ensure that segmentation performance does not degrade regardless of which modality is missing. We propose a new architecture and learning method for building a robust "single" model in all missing modality scenarios.

**Scenario-Specific Fusion (SsF) Decoders.** To achieve robust segmentation performance in any scenario, the model must learn representations from the full modality scenario which is the most informative. However, it is difficult for a single fusion decoder to continue learning representations from the full modality scenario. Therefore, in this section, we expand a single fusion decoder into three

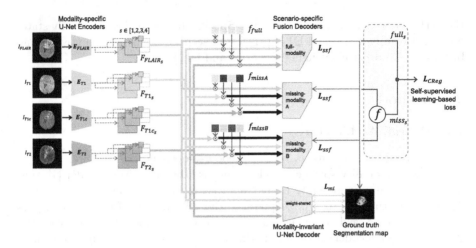

**Fig. 1.** Overall architecture. $F_{FLAIR_s}$ means the four feature maps that output each modality-specific encoder for the modality $FLAIR$ and stage $s \in [1,2,3,4]$. The notations are the same with the other modalities $T1, T1c$ and $T2$. The feature maps for the modalities undergo scenario-specific fusion (SsF) decoders, preceded by specialized binary code filters $f_{full}, f_{missA}, f_{missB}$ for each SSF decoder.

scenario-specific fusion (SsF) decoders that fuse distinctive feature maps for each input scenario.

As shown in Fig. 1, three SsF decoders consist of two missing-modality SsF decoders and one full-modality SsF decoder. Each missing-modality SsF decoder learns representations for mutually exclusive scenarios. We will explain why we deal with mutually exclusive scenarios in the next "Self-supervised learning-based loss" part. Of course, the full-modality SsF decoder learns representations for the full-modality scenario. The full-modality SsF decoder plays a strong supervision role to ensure that two missing-modality SsF decoders, can sufficiently learn information from the full-modality scenario. For easier understanding, we will use the subscript (or superscript) notations $missA$ and $missB$ for the two missing-modality SsF decoders, and $full$ for the full-modality SsF decoder.

As we mentioned earlier, each modality-specific encoder outputs four feature maps $[F_{m_1}, F_{m_2}, F_{m_3}, F_{m_4}]$ for each modality $m$. After encoding, each SsF decoder filters the feature maps from all modalities with its own independent filter. The filters for the missing-modality SsF decoders $f_{missA}$ and $f_{missB}$ are determined by binary codes that express the presence or absence of each modality. Meanwhile, the filter for the full-modality SsF decoder $f_{full}$ is the same regardless of the binary code. For each $s \in [1,2,3,4]$, the final inputs for three SsF decoders are as follows:

$$[F_{FLAIR_s}^{full}, F_{T1_s}^{full}, F_{T1c_s}^{full}, F_{T2_s}^{full}] = f_{full} \otimes [F_{FLAIR_s}, F_{T1_s}, F_{T1c_s}, F_{T2_s}], \quad (2)$$

$$[F^{missA}_{FLAIR_s}, F^{missA}_{T1_s}, F^{missA}_{T1c_s}, F^{missA}_{T2_s}] = f_{missA} \otimes [F_{FLAIR_s}, F_{T1_s}, F_{T1c_s}, F_{T2_s}],$$
(3)
$$[F^{missB}_{FLAIR_s}, F^{missB}_{T1_s}, F^{missB}_{T1c_s}, F^{missB}_{T2_s}] = f_{missB} \otimes [F_{FLAIR_s}, F_{T1_s}, F_{T1c_s}, F_{T2_s}],$$
(4)

where $\otimes$ means *matmul* operation between two tensors. Each SsF decoder fuses four final inputs and then outputs intermediate feature maps for each stage and predicted segmentation map. The structure of the fusion decoder utilizes the U-Net decoder and attention-based fusion [5].

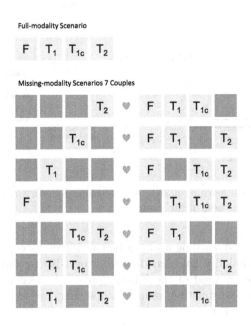

**Fig. 2.** The self-evident fact is used to define new loss function $\mathcal{L}_{CReg}$ based on self-supervised learning: In 14 missing-modality scenarios, each couple produces one full-modality scenario when they are added together.

**Self-supervised Learning-based loss: Couple Regularization (CReg).** To sufficiently learn the representation in the full modality scenario, We find the new self-evident fact which is specialized in missing modality brain tumor segmentation field. In this section, we define a new loss function based on self-supervised learning that uses the self-evident fact that has never been used for missing modality model training. As shown in Fig. 2, there are the 15 scenarios of missing modality brain tumor segmentation, 14 scenarios excluding full modality can be paired two by two and become full modality when they are added together. For example, a scenario with only T2 missing is paired with a scenario where all modalities except T2 are missing. Based on this simple but strong fact, we propose a novel self-supervised learning-based loss function to train a total of three SsF decoder models, two for the missing-modality scenarios and one for the full-modality scenario. For this, we first named the prediction of each SsF decoder and fusion block with $full_s$, $missA_s$, and $missB_s$ like the right side of Fig. 1. Then we can define the task that makes the $miss_s = f(missA_s, missB_s)$ to learn a representation as similar as possible to $full_s$, where $s \in [1, 2, 3, 4]$ as shown in Fig. 3.

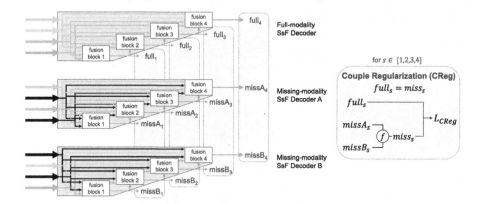

**Fig. 3.** Self-supervised learning-based loss function named Couple Regularization $\mathcal{L}_{CReg}$ to improve robustness of the model.

This self-supervised learning also can be considered as regularization to prevent two missing-modality SsF decoders from over-fitting during training and to follow the fusion method of the full-modality SsF decoder well. Therefore, we proposed a new loss function named Couple Regularization (CReg) $\mathcal{L}_{CReg}$, "Couple" means pair of scenarios:

$$\mathcal{L}_{CReg} = \sum_s \mathcal{L}(miss_s, full_s), \tag{5}$$

where $miss_s = f(missA_s, missB_s)$ and $s \in [1, 2, 3, 4]$. A function $f$ means deconvolution after concatenation. The proposed loss $\mathcal{L}_{CReg}$ consists of two types of losses, a weighted cross-entropy loss $\mathcal{L}_{WCE}$ [5] and a Dice loss $\mathcal{L}_{Dice}$ [11].

$$\mathcal{L}(X, Y) = \mathcal{L}_{WCE}(X, Y) + \mathcal{L}_{Dice}(X, Y), \tag{6}$$

$$\mathcal{L}_{WCE}(X, Y) = \sum_{r \in R} \frac{|| - \alpha_r \cdot Y_r \cdot log(X_r)||_1}{H \cdot W \cdot Z}, \tag{7}$$

where $\alpha_r = 1 - \frac{||Y_r||_1}{\sum_{r' \in R} ||Y_{r'}||_1}$ is the weight for the key tumor region $r \in R = \{$ background, NCR-NET, ED, ET$\}$.

$$\mathcal{L}_{Dice}(X, Y) = 1 - \frac{2 \cdot \sum_{r \in R} \sum_i^{V_r} X_i Y_i}{\sum_{r \in R} \sum_i^{V_r} X_i^2 + \sum_{r \in R} \sum_i^{V_r} Y_i^2}, \tag{8}$$

where $V_r$ is the number of voxels in region $r \in R$.

## 2.3   Lifelong Learning Strategy (LLS)

To achieve robust segmentation performance in any scenario, it is important not only to sufficiently learn the representation in the most informative scenario but also not to forget the learned information even after the training ends. In this regard, we propose a Lifelong Learning Strategy that prevents two missing-modality SsF decoders from forgetting the rich representation in the full-modality scenario during training. We use a different combination of SsF decoders from the one proposed above in the initial training epochs and iterations. Specifically, during the initial epochs (smaller than $epoch_{lls}$) and iterations (smaller than $iter_{lls}$) where the lifelong-learning strategy is applied, we replace all SsF decoders with full-modality SsF decoders. $epoch_{lls}$ and $iter_{lls}$ are controlled as hyperparameters. In this way, the two missing-modality decoders can continuously learn the representation in the full-modality scenario during training, and the missing-modality segmentation performance can be improved as much as in the full-modality scenario.

## 2.4   Total Loss

$$\mathcal{L}_{total} = \mathcal{L}_{ssf} + \mathcal{L}_{mi} + \lambda_{CReg}\mathcal{L}_{CReg} \tag{9}$$

The total loss function for training the 4-encoder-4-decoder architecture including Scenario-specific Fusion (SsF) decoders with newly defined self-supervised learning-based loss function, named couple regularization $\mathcal{L}_{CReg}$. $\lambda_{CReg}$ is a hyperparameter and $\mathcal{L}_{ssf}$ and $\mathcal{L}_{mi}$ are for comparing the outputs of scenario-specific fusion decoder and modality-invariant U-Net decoder, respectively. All three losses are composed of $\mathcal{L}_{WCE}$ and $\mathcal{L}_{Dice}$ as described earlier.

$$\mathcal{L}_{ssf} = \sum_{s} \mathcal{L}_s(\hat{y}_s, y), \tag{10}$$

$$\mathcal{L}_{mi} = \sum_{m} \mathcal{L}_m(\hat{y}_m, y), \tag{11}$$

where $\hat{y}_s$ is the result of each fusion block for $s \in [1, 2, 3, 4]$, and $\hat{y}_m$ is for $m \in \{FLAIR, T1c, T1, T2\}$ is modality, and $y$ is ground-truth mask.

# 3   Experimental Results

## 3.1   Experimental Setup

**Dataset.** BraTS2018 (Brain Tumor Segmentation Challenge 2018) [10] contains MRI scans of 285 patients with gliomas, a type of brain tumor. The scans include four different modalities: T1-weighted (T1), T1-weighted with contrast enhancement (T1c), T2-weighted (T2), and FLAIR. The BraTS2018 training dataset includes 210 patient MRI scans, along with their corresponding segmentation labels. We use the same split lists as in [6]. For each patient, the dataset includes ground truth segmentation labels for three tumor sub-regions: the whole tumor (WT), the tumor core (TC), and the enhancing tumor (ET). The WT label in the BraTS dataset includes all three key tumor regions: the necrotic and non-enhancing tumor core (NCR/NET), the peritumoral edema (ED), and the enhancing tumor (ET). The TC label is composed of NCR/NET and ET, while the ET label is comprised only of the ET. The key tumor regions are segmented based on different modalities.

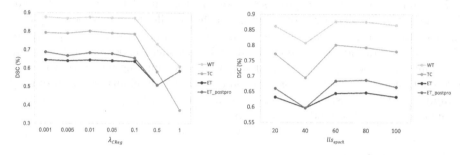

**Fig. 4.** (left) Hyperparameter $\lambda_{CReg}$ tuning. (right) Hyperparameter $lls_{epoch}$ tuning.

**Implementation and Evaluation.** We followed the same pre-processing step as in [3,5,6], which includes skull-stripping, co-registration, re-sampling to a resolution $1mm^3$, removal of the black background outside the brain, and zero-mean and unit-variance normalization using values of the brain area. During training, the input images are randomly cropped to $80 \times 80 \times 80$. Data augmentation is also applied using random rotations, intensity shifts, and mirror flipping. We train the proposed model for 300 epochs with 50 iterations per epoch and the batch size is 1. Adam optimizer is used with $\beta_1$ and $\beta_2$ set to 0.9 and 0.999, respectively. Weight decay is set to $1e^{-5}$, and a learning rate scheduler that reduces the learning rate by a factor of $(1 - \frac{epoch}{max_{epoch}})^{0.9}$ is adopted. Moreover, Fig. 4 presents the experimental results conducted by varying the hyperparameters in the full-modality scenario. Based on the results, we selected hyperparameters $epoch_{lls}, iter_{lls}, \lambda_{CReg}$ as 60, 10, and 0.01, respectively. The segmentation performance was evaluated using the Dice Similarity Coefficient (DSC) metric for three brain tumor sub-regions in each scenario.

### 3.2   Results and Analysis

**Comparisons with SOTA Models.** We compare our model RobustSsF with three state-of-the-art methods: one "dedicated" model ACN [14] and two "single" models RF-Net [5] and MFI [17]. Table 1 shows that our proposed model achieves state-of-the-art (SOTA) performance in terms of average and standard deviation for all 15 scenarios. In particular, RobustSsF demonstrated remarkable performance in terms of standard deviation. Regardless of the type of model used for comparison, **ours successfully reduces the standard deviations** - from 12 times lower in Whole Tumor to 76 times lower in Enhancing Tumor. A low standard deviation indicates that the performance gap between the scenarios for the model is low, which means that the model demonstrates robust performance across all scenarios. When comparing performance results directly, other models experience up to a 54% decrease in performance from Scenario 1 to Scenario 15 for the most difficult ET sub-region. However, RobustSsF exhibits only a **0.8% difference** in performance between these two scenarios. Moreover, **ours also achieves the best performance in all scenarios where T1ce modality**

**Table 1.** Comparisons with SOTA models including one "dedicated" model ACN [14] and two "single" models RF-Net [5] and MFI [17] on BraTS2018. The results were obtained either by directly extracting them from the papers or by reproducing the authors' code. The last column is the result of applying post-processing [5] to the ET label.

| | | Scenarios | | | Whole Tumor (WT) | | | | Tumor Core (TC) | | | | Enhancing Tumor (ET) | | | | ET_postpro | |
|---|---|---|---|---|---|---|---|---|---|---|---|---|---|---|---|---|---|---|
| # | F | T1 | T1c | T2 | ACN | RFNet | MFI | Ours | ACN | RFNet | MFI | Ours | ACN | RFNet | MFI | Ours | RFNet | Ours |
| 1 | ○ | ○ | ○ | ● | 85.55 | 85.41 | 85.63 | **87.65** | 67.94 | 69.25 | 67.48 | **79.53** | 42.98 | 43.71 | 37.42 | **64.34** | 47.55 | **67.85** |
| 2 | ○ | ○ | ● | ○ | 80.52 | 75.17 | 75.24 | **87.27** | 84.18 | 81.34 | 80.90 | 80.33 | 78.07 | 69.76 | 76.19 | 64.44 | 73.11 | 67.68 |
| 3 | ○ | ● | ○ | ○ | 79.34 | 73.90 | 74.23 | **87.13** | 71.18 | 61.41 | 63.13 | **78.78** | 41.52 | 33.32 | 32.28 | **64.34** | 35.23 | **67.84** |
| 4 | ● | ○ | ○ | ○ | 87.30 | 86.82 | 86.42 | **87.37** | 67.72 | 69.09 | 63.72 | **79.48** | 42.77 | 37.05 | 37.63 | **64.35** | 38.75 | **69.25** |
| 5 | ○ | ○ | ● | ● | 86.41 | 87.11 | 86.52 | **87.58** | 84.41 | **84.56** | 84.03 | 80.66 | 75.65 | 72.83 | **77.56** | 64.18 | **76.29** | 67.69 |
| 6 | ○ | ● | ● | ○ | 80.05 | 79.58 | 78.65 | **87.62** | **84.59** | 83.26 | 81.92 | 80.60 | 75.21 | 73.20 | **76.78** | 64.67 | 74.26 | 67.82 |
| 7 | ● | ● | ○ | ○ | 87.49 | 89.29 | **89.52** | 87.56 | 71.30 | 72.21 | 72.74 | **79.42** | 43.71 | 39.75 | 41.34 | **63.95** | 45.63 | **69.21** |
| 8 | ○ | ● | ○ | ● | 85.50 | 87.37 | 86.56 | **87.64** | 73.28 | 72.82 | 71.41 | **79.32** | 47.39 | 45.28 | 41.37 | **63.99** | 47.23 | **67.5** |
| 9 | ● | ○ | ○ | ● | 87.75 | 89.60 | **90.04** | 87.58 | 71.61 | 72.67 | 71.28 | **79.89** | 45.96 | 45.75 | 42.52 | **64.43** | 49.47 | **67.94** |
| 10 | ● | ○ | ● | ○ | 88.28 | 89.44 | **89.99** | 87.74 | 83.35 | 84.60 | **84.65** | 80.16 | 77.46 | 71.80 | **78.79** | 64.32 | **75.10** | 67.82 |
| 11 | ● | ● | ● | ○ | 88.96 | **90.12** | 90.11 | 87.97 | 84.25 | 84.98 | **85.16** | 80.46 | 76.16 | 72.76 | **79.81** | 64.71 | **77.07** | 68.22 |
| 12 | ● | ● | ○ | ● | 88.35 | **90.41** | 90.33 | 87.54 | 67.86 | 74.58 | 73.95 | **80.01** | 42.09 | 46.33 | 43.42 | **64.44** | 50.21 | **67.95** |
| 13 | ● | ○ | ● | ● | 88.34 | 90.14 | **90.80** | 87.80 | 82.85 | 84.78 | **85.51** | 80.46 | 75.97 | 72.39 | **79.41** | 64.24 | **75.52** | 69.51 |
| 14 | ○ | ● | ● | ● | 86.90 | **87.91** | 86.94 | 87.78 | 84.67 | **85.01** | 84.13 | 80.49 | 76.10 | 73.20 | **77.91** | 64.83 | **76.48** | 69.59 |
| 15 | ● | ● | ● | ● | 89.22 | 90.76 | **90.88** | 88.34 | 85.18 | 85.35 | **85.63** | 81.46 | 77.06 | 72.86 | **79.98** | 64.90 | **77.15** | 69.80 |
| | | Average ↑ | | | 86.00 | 86.20 | 86.12 | **87.638** | 77.62 | 77.72 | 77.04 | **80.07** | 61.21 | 57.99 | 60.16 | **64.41** | 61.27 | **68.38** |
| | | Std ↓ | | | 3.311 | 5.316 | 5.587 | **0.2766** | 7.426 | 7.544 | 8.291 | **0.6553** | 16.95 | 15.68 | 20.26 | **0.2667** | 15.78 | **0.7978** |

**Table 2.** Ablation study. DSC (%). SsF means Scenario-specific Fusion.

| | | WT | TC | ET |
|---|---|---|---|---|
| Only one fusion decoder (baseline) | average ↑ | 86.20 | 77.73 | 58.00 |
| | std ↓ | 5.316 | 7.545 | 15.68 |
| + $\mathcal{L}_{CReg}$ only for final prediction with three SsF decoders | average ↑ | 85.49 | 75.80 | 62.66 |
| | std ↓ | 0.1500 | 0.2484 | 0.3152 |
| + Lifelong Learning Strategy (LLS) | average ↑ | 87.46 | **80.46** | **65.07** |
| | std ↓ | 0.2521 | 0.5226 | 0.9104 |
| + $\mathcal{L}_{CReg}$ all outputs | average ↑ | **87.64** | 80.07 | 64.41 |
| | std ↓ | 0.2767 | 0.6553 | 0.2668 |

**is missing,** 1,3,4,7,8,9,12th scenarios (row) in Table 1. As a result, we have successfully created a more robust network compared to existing state-of-the-art methods in missing modality brain tumor segmentation.

**Ablation Study.** To validate the effects of each important component of our proposed model, we evaluate the performance by adding each component one by one to the baseline. As shown in Table 2, even by expanding one decoder to three and applying the newly defined self-supervised learning-based loss function named couple regularization only to the final prediction, the standard deviation dramatically decreases. This indicates that our Scenario-specific Fusion (SsF) decoders with self-supervised learning-based loss function $\mathcal{L}_{CReg}$ play a crucial role in improving the model's robustness. In addition, we can observe that Lifelong Learning Strategy (LLS) improves the performance without losing the model's robustness. Finally, applying $\mathcal{L}_{CReg}$ to the intermediate outputs of SsF decoders also slightly improves the performance and helps build a more robust model.

## 4    Conclusion

In this paper, we propose a novel MRI brain tumor segmentation model, called RobustSsF which incorporates scenario-specific fusion decoders with self-supervised learning and newly defined couple regularization loss. Our model outperforms state-of-the-art methods in terms of average accuracy and standard deviation on the BraTS2018 dataset, even in all scenarios where the T1ce modality is missing which is hard to collect compared to the other three modalities. Based on the quantitative results, we successfully improved robustness to handle all missing modality scenarios, which makes it a promising approach for clinical applications. Future work could include extending our approach to handle other medical image segmentation tasks or exploring the use of more advanced self-supervised learning techniques.

**Acknowledgements.** This work was supported by the Engineering Research Center of Excellence (ERC) Program supported by National Research Foundation (NRF), Korean Ministry of Science & ICT (MSIT) (Grant No. NRF-2017R1A5A101470823).

## References

1. Azad, R., Khosravi, N., Dehghanmanshadi, M., Cohen-Adad, J., Merhof, D.: Medical image segmentation on MRI images with missing modalities: a review (2022)
2. Azad, R., Khosravi, N., Merhof, D.: SMU-net: style matching U-net for brain tumor segmentation with missing modalities (2022)
3. Chen, C., Dou, Q., Jin, Y., Chen, H., Qin, J., Heng, P.A.: Robust multimodal brain tumor segmentation via feature disentanglement and gated fusion (2020)

4. Çiçek, Ö., Abdulkadir, A., Lienkamp, S.S., Brox, T., Ronneberger, O.: 3D U-net: learning dense volumetric segmentation from sparse annotation. In: Ourselin, S., Joskowicz, L., Sabuncu, M.R., Unal, G., Wells, W. (eds.) MICCAI 2016. LNCS, vol. 9901, pp. 424–432. Springer, Cham (2016). https://doi.org/10.1007/978-3-319-46723-8_49

5. Ding, Y., Yu, X., Yang, Y.: RFnet: region-aware fusion network for incomplete multi-modal brain tumor segmentation. In: 2021 IEEE/CVF International Conference on Computer Vision (ICCV), pp. 3955–3964 (2021)

6. Dorent, R., Joutard, S., Modat, M., Ourselin, S., Vercauteren, T.: Hetero-modal variational encoder-decoder for joint modality completion and segmentation. In: Shen, D., et al. (eds.) MICCAI 2019. LNCS, vol. 11765, pp. 74–82. Springer, Cham (2019). https://doi.org/10.1007/978-3-030-32245-8_9

7. Havaei, M., Guizard, N., Chapados, N., Bengio, Y.: Hemis: hetero-modal image segmentation. CoRR abs/1607.05194 (2016)

8. Hu, M., et al.: Knowledge distillation from multi-modal to mono-modal segmentation networks (2021)

9. Li, Z., Hoiem, D.: Learning without forgetting (2016)

10. Menze, B.H., et al.: The multimodal brain tumor image segmentation benchmark (brats). IEEE Trans. Med. Imaging **34**(10), 1993–2024 (2015). https://doi.org/10.1109/TMI.2014.2377694

11. Milletari, F., Navab, N., Ahmadi, S.A.: V-net: Fully convolutional neural networks for volumetric medical image segmentation (2016)

12. Serrà, J., Surís, D., Miron, M., Karatzoglou, A.: Overcoming catastrophic forgetting with hard attention to the task (2018)

13. Shin, H., Lee, J.K., Kim, J., Kim, J.: Continual learning with deep generative replay (2017)

14. Wang, Y., et al.: ACN: adversarial co-training network for brain tumor segmentation with missing modalities (2021)

15. Yoon, J., Yang, E., Lee, J., Hwang, S.J.: Lifelong learning with dynamically expandable networks (2017)

16. Zhang, Y., et al.: mmformer: Multimodal medical transformer for incomplete multimodal learning of brain tumor segmentation (2022)

17. Zhao, Z., Yang, H., Sun, J.: Modality-adaptive feature interaction for brain tumor segmentation with missing modalities. In: Wang, L., Dou, Q., Fletcher, P.T., Speidel, S., Li, S. (eds.) MICCAI 2022. LNCS, vol. 13435, pp. 183–192. Springer, Cham (2022). https://doi.org/10.1007/978-3-031-16443-9_18

18. Zhou, T., Ruan, S., Hu, H.: A literature survey of MR-based brain tumor segmentation with missing modalities. Comput. Med. Imaging Graph. **104**, 102167 (2023)

# Semi-supervised Cooperative Learning for Multiomics Data Fusion

Daisy Yi Ding[(✉)], Xiaotao Shen, Michael Snyder, and Robert Tibshirani

Stanford University, Stanford, CA 94305, USA
dingd@stanford.edu

**Abstract.** Multiomics data fusion integrates diverse data modalities, ranging from transcriptomics to proteomics, to gain a comprehensive understanding of biological systems and enhance predictions on outcomes of interest related to disease phenotypes and treatment responses. Cooperative learning, a recently proposed method, unifies the commonly-used fusion approaches, including early and late fusion, and offers a systematic framework for leveraging the shared underlying relationships across omics to strengthen signals. However, the challenge of acquiring large-scale labeled data remains, and there are cases where multiomics data are available but in the absence of annotated labels. To harness the potential of unlabeled multiomcis data, we introduce semi-supervised cooperative learning. By utilizing an "agreement penalty", our method incorporates the additional unlabeled data in the learning process and achieves consistently superior predictive performance on simulated data and a real multiomics study of aging. It offers an effective solution to multiomics data fusion in settings with both labeled and unlabeled data and maximizes the utility of available data resources, with the potential of significantly improving predictive models for diagnostics and therapeutics in an increasingly multiomics world.

**Keywords:** Multiomics data fusion · Semi-supervised learning · Machine learning

## 1 Introduction

With advancements in biotechnologies, significant progress has been made in generating and collecting a diverse range of "-omics" data on a common set of patients, including genomics, epigenomics, transcriptomics, proteomics, and metabolomics (Fig. 1A). These data characterize molecular variations of human health from different perspectives and of different granularities. Fusing the multiple data modalities on a common set of observations provides the opportunity to gain a more holistic understanding of outcomes of interest such as disease phenotypes and treatment response. It offers the potential to discover hidden insights that may remain obscured in single-modality data analyses and achieve more accurate predictions of the outcomes [13,14,16,18,20,21]. While the term

© The Author(s), under exclusive license to Springer Nature Switzerland AG 2024
A. K. Maier et al. (Eds.): ML4MHD 2023, LNCS 14315, pp. 54–63, 2024.
https://doi.org/10.1007/978-3-031-47679-2_5

"multiomics data fusion" can have various interpretations, we use it here in the context of predicting an outcome of interest by integrating different data modalities.

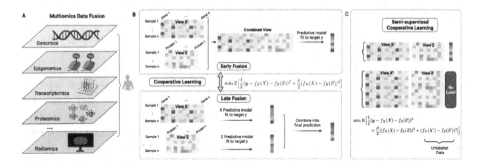

**Fig. 1.** *Framework of semi-supervised cooperative learning for multiomics data fusion.* *(A)* The advancements in biotechnologies have led to the generation and collection of diverse "omics" data on a common set of samples, ranging from genomics to proteomics. Fusing the data provides a unique opportunity to gain a holistic understanding of complex biological systems and enhance predictive accuracy on outcomes of interest related to disease phenotypes and treatment response *(B)* Commonly-used approaches to multiomics data fusion have two broad categories: early fusion involves transforming all data modalities into a unified representation before feeding it into a model of choice, while late fusion builds separate models for each data modality and combines their predictions using a second-level model. Encompassing early and late fusion, cooperative learning exploits the shared underlying relationships across omics for enhanced predictive performance. *(C)* The field of biomedicine faces a persistent challenge due to the scarcity of large-scale labeled data, which requires significant resources to acquire. In cases where unlabeled multiomics data are also accessible, we introduce semi-supervised cooperative learning to leverage the combined information from both labeled and unlabeled data. The agreement penalty seamlessly integrates the unlabeled samples into the learning process, effectively utilizing the shared underlying signals present in both labeled and unlabeled data and maximizing the utility of available data resources for multiomics data fusion.

Commonly-used data fusion methods can be broadly categorized into early and late fusion (Fig. 1*B*). Early fusion works by transforming the multiple data modalities into a single representation before feeding the aggregated representation into a supervised learning model of choice [4,11,19,26]. Late fusion refers to methods where individual models are first built from the distinct data modality, and then the predictions of the individual models are combined into the final predictor [3,5,24,25,27]. However, both methods do not explicitly leverage the shared underlying relationship across modalities, and a systematic framework for multiomics data fusion is lacking.

To tackle this limitation, a new method called *cooperative learning* has recently been proposed [8]. It combines the usual squared error loss of predictions with an "agreement" penalty to encourage alignment of predictions from different data modalities (Fig. 1 *B*). By varying the weight of the agreement penalty, one can get a continuum of solutions that include early and late fusion. Cooperative learning chooses the degree of fusion in a data-adaptive manner, providing enhanced flexibility and performance. It has demonstrated effectiveness on both simulated data and real multiomics data, particularly when the different data modalities share some underlying relationships in their signals that can be exploited to boost the signals.

However, an important challenge persists in the field of biomedicine: the scarcity of large-scale labeled data. Acquiring a substantial amount of labeled data in this domain often demands considerable effort, time, and financial resources. Nonetheless, there are instances where multiomics data are available, but in the absence of corresponding labels. In such cases, it becomes imperative to leverage the available unlabeled data to enhance predictive models.

To harness the potential of unlabeled data, we propose *semi-supervised cooperative learning*. The key idea is to utilize the agreement penalty, inherent in the cooperative learning framework, as a means to leverage the matched unlabeled samples to our advantage (Fig. 1 *C*). It acts as a mechanism for incorporating the unlabeled samples into the learning process, by encouraging the predictions from different data modalities to align not only on the labeled samples but also on the unlabeled ones. Semi-supervised cooperative learning leverages the additional shared underlying signals across the unlabeled data and exploits the valuable information that would otherwise remain untapped. Through comprehensive simulated studies and a real multiomics study of aging, we showed that our method achieves consistently higher predictive accuracy on the outcomes of interest. By incorporating matched unlabeled data and thus maximizing the utility of available data, semi-supervised cooperative learning offers an effective solution to multiomics data fusion, with the potential to significantly enhance predictive models and unlock hidden insights in health and disease.

## 2    Approach

### 2.1    Cooperative Learning

We begin by giving a concise overview of the recently proposed *cooperative learning* framework [8] to set the stage for the introduction of *semi-supervised cooperative learning*. Let $X \in \mathcal{R}^{n \times p_x}$, $Z \in \mathcal{R}^{n \times p_z}$ — representing two data views — and $y \in \mathcal{R}^n$ be a real-valued response. Fixing the hyperparameter $\rho \geq 0$, cooperative learning aims to minimize the population quantity:

$$\min \mathrm{E}\left[\frac{1}{2}(y - f_X(X) - f_Z(Z))^2 + \frac{\rho}{2}(f_X(X) - f_Z(Z))^2\right]. \tag{1}$$

The first term is the usual prediction error loss, while the second term is an "agreement" penalty, encouraging alignment of predictions from different modalities.

To be more concrete in the setting of regularized linear regression, for a fixed value of the hyperparameter $\rho \geq 0$, cooperative learning finds $\boldsymbol{\theta_x} \in \mathcal{R}^{p_x}$ and $\boldsymbol{\theta_z} \in \mathcal{R}^{p_z}$ that minimize:

$$J(\boldsymbol{\theta_x}, \boldsymbol{\theta_z}) = \frac{1}{2}||\boldsymbol{y} - X\boldsymbol{\theta_x} - Z\boldsymbol{\theta_z}||^2 + \frac{\rho}{2}||(X\boldsymbol{\theta_x} - Z\boldsymbol{\theta_z})||^2$$
$$+\lambda_x||\boldsymbol{\theta_x}||_1 + \lambda_z||\boldsymbol{\theta_z}||_1. \quad (2)$$

where $\rho$ is the hyperparameter that controls the relative importance of the agreement penalty term $||(X\boldsymbol{\theta_x} - Z\boldsymbol{\theta_z})||^2$ in the objective, and $\lambda_x||\boldsymbol{\theta_x}||_1$ and $\lambda_z||\boldsymbol{\theta_z}||_1$ are $\ell_1$ penalties[1].

When $\rho = 0$, cooperative learning reduces to early fusion, where we simply use the combined set of features in a supervised learning procedure. When $\rho = 1$, we can show that it yields a simple form of late fusion. In addition, theoretical analysis has demonstrated that the agreement penalty offers an advantage in reducing the mean-squared error of the predictions under a latent factor model [8].

## 2.2 Semi-supervised Cooperative Learning

In this section, we present *semi-supervised cooperative learning*, which enables us to harness the power of both labeled and unlabeled data for multiomics data fusion. Consider feature matrices $X \in \mathcal{R}^{n \times p_x}$, $Z \in \mathcal{R}^{n \times p_z}$, with labels $\boldsymbol{y} \in \mathcal{R}^n$, and then additional feature matrices $X' \in \mathcal{R}^{n_{\text{unlabeled}} \times p_x}$, $Z' \in \mathcal{R}^{n_{\text{unlabeled}} \times p_z}$, without labels. The objective of semi-supervised cooperative learning is

$$\min \mathrm{E}\left[\frac{1}{2}(\boldsymbol{y} - f_X(X) - f_Z(Z))^2 + \frac{\rho}{2}[(f_X(X) - f_Z(Z))^2 + (f_X(X') - f_Z(Z'))^2]\right].$$
$$(3)$$

The agreement penalty allows us to use the matched unlabeled samples to our advantage, by encouraging predictions from different data modalities to align on both labeled and unlabeled samples, thus leveraging the aligned signals across omics in a semi-supervised manner. This agreement penalty term is also related to "contrastive learning" [6,15], which is an unsupervised learning technique first proposed for learning visual representations. Without the supervision of $\boldsymbol{y}$, it learns representations of images by maximizing agreement between differently augmented "views" of the same data example. While contrastive learning is unsupervised and cooperative learning is supervised, both of which have a term in the objective that encourages agreement between correlated views, semi-supervised cooperative learning combines the strengths of both paradigms to fully exploit labeled and unlabeled data simultaneously.

---

[1] We assume that the columns of $X$ and $Z$ have been standardized, and $\boldsymbol{y}$ has mean 0 (hence we can omit the intercept). We use the commonly-used $\ell_1$ penalties for illustration, while the framework generalizes to other penalty functions.

In the regularized regression setting and with a common $\lambda^2$, the objective becomes

$$J(\boldsymbol{\theta}_x, \boldsymbol{\theta}_z) = \frac{1}{2}||\boldsymbol{y} - X\boldsymbol{\theta}_x - Z\boldsymbol{\theta}_z||^2 + \frac{\rho}{2}[||(X\boldsymbol{\theta}_x - Z\boldsymbol{\theta}_z)||^2 + ||(X'\boldsymbol{\theta}_x - Z'\boldsymbol{\theta}_z)||^2]$$
$$+ \lambda(||\boldsymbol{\theta}_x||_1 + ||\boldsymbol{\theta}_z||_1), \quad (4)$$

and one can compute a regularization path of solutions indexed by $\lambda$. Problem (4) is convex, and the solution can be computed as follows. Letting

$$\tilde{X} = \begin{pmatrix} X & Z \\ -\sqrt{\rho}X & \sqrt{\rho}Z \\ -\sqrt{\rho}X' & \sqrt{\rho}Z' \end{pmatrix}, \tilde{y} = \begin{pmatrix} \boldsymbol{y} \\ 0 \\ 0 \end{pmatrix}, \tilde{\beta} = \begin{pmatrix} \boldsymbol{\theta}_x \\ \boldsymbol{\theta}_z \end{pmatrix}, \quad (5)$$

then the equivalent problem to (4) is

$$\frac{1}{2}||\tilde{y} - \tilde{X}\tilde{\beta}||^2 + \lambda(||\boldsymbol{\theta}_x||_1 + ||\boldsymbol{\theta}_z||_1). \quad (6)$$

This is a form of the lasso, and can be computed, for example by the `glmnet` package [9].

Let $\text{Lasso}(X, \boldsymbol{y}, \lambda)$ denote the generic problem:

$$\min_\beta \frac{1}{2}||\boldsymbol{y} - X\beta||^2 + \lambda||\beta||_1. \quad (7)$$

We outline the algorithm for semi-supervised cooperative learning in Algorithm 1.

---

**Algorithm 1.** *Semi-supervised cooperative learning.*

---

**Input:** $X \in \mathcal{R}^{n \times p_x}$ and $Z \in \mathcal{R}^{n \times p_z}$, the response $\boldsymbol{y} \in \mathcal{R}^n$, and the unlabeled data $X' \in \mathcal{R}^{n_{\text{unlabeled}} \times p_x}$ and $Z' \in \mathcal{R}^{n_{\text{unlabeled}} \times p_z}$, and a grid of hyperparameter values $(\rho_{\min}, \ldots, \rho_{\max})$.

**for** $\rho \leftarrow \rho_{\min}, \ldots, \rho_{\max}$ **do**

Set

$$\tilde{X} = \begin{pmatrix} X & Z \\ -\sqrt{\rho}X & \sqrt{\rho}Z \\ -\sqrt{\rho}X' & \sqrt{\rho}Z' \end{pmatrix}, \tilde{y} = \begin{pmatrix} \boldsymbol{y} \\ 0 \\ 0 \end{pmatrix}.$$

Solve $\text{Lasso}(\tilde{X}, \tilde{y}, \lambda)$ over a decreasing grid of $\lambda$ values.

**end**

Select the optimal value of $\rho^*$ based on the CV error and get the final fit.

---

---

$^2$ It was shown in [8] that there is generally no advantage to allowing different $\lambda$ values for different modalities.

# 3   Experiments

## 3.1   Simulated Studies

We first compare semi-supervised cooperative learning with vanilla cooperative learning, early and late fusion methods in simulation studies. We generated Gaussian data with $n = 200$ and $p = 500$ in each of two views $X$ and $Z$, and created correlation between them using latent factors. The response $y$ was generated as

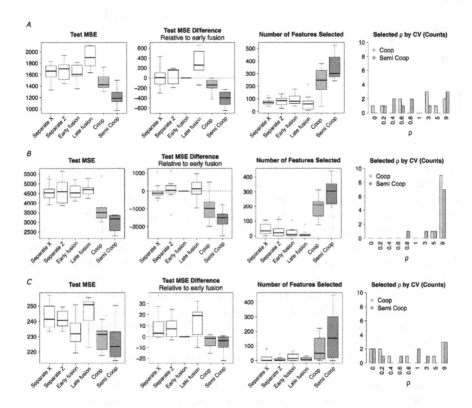

**Fig. 2.** *Simulation studies on semi-supervised cooperative learning. (A) Simulation results when $X$ I $Z$ have a medium level of correlation ($t = 2, s_u = 1$); both $X$ and $Z$ contain signal ($b_x = b_z = 2$), $n = 200, n_{\mathrm{unlabel}} = 200, p = 1000$, SNR = 1.8. The first panel shows MSE on a test set; the second panel shows the MSE difference on the test set relative to early fusion; the third panel shows the number of features selected; the fourth panel shows the $\rho$ values selected by CV in cooperative learning and semi-supervised cooperative learning. Here "Coop" refers to cooperative learning and "Semi Coop" refers to semi-supervised cooperative learning. (B) Simulation results when $X$ and $Z$ have a high level of correlation ($t = 6, s_u = 1$); only $X$ contains signal ($b_x = 2, b_z = 0$), $n = 200, n_{\mathrm{unlabel}} = 200, p = 1000$, SNR = 0.5. (C) Simulation results when $X$ and $Z$ have no correlation ($t = 0, s_u = 1$); both $X$ and $Z$ contain signal ($b_x = b_z = 2$), $n = 200, n_{\mathrm{unlabel}} = 200, p = 1000$, SNR = 1.0.*

a linear combination of the latent factors, corrupted by Gaussian noise. We then generated an additional set of unlabeled data $X'$ and $Z'$ with $n_{\text{unlabeled}} = 200$ and $p = 500$.

The simulation is set up as follows. Given values for parameters $n, n_{\text{unlabled}}, p_x, p_z, p_u, s_u, t_x, t_z, \beta_u, \sigma$, we generate data according to the following procedure:

1. $x_j \in \mathcal{R}^n$ and $x'_j \in \mathcal{R}^n$ distributed i.i.d. MVN$(0, I_n)$ for $j = 1, 2, \ldots, p_x$.
2. $z_j \in \mathcal{R}^n$ and $z'_j \in \mathcal{R}^n$ distributed i.i.d. MVN$(0, I_n)$ for $j = 1, 2, \ldots, p_z$.
3. For $i = 1, 2, \ldots, p_u$ ($p_u$ corresponds to the number of latent factors, $p_u < p_x$ and $p_u < p_z$):
   (a) $u_i \in \mathcal{R}^n$ and $u'_i \in \mathcal{R}^n$ distributed i.i.d. MVN$(0, s_u^2 I_n)$;
   (b) $x_i = x_i + t_x * u_i$,    $x'_i = x'_i + t_x * u'_i$;
   (c) $z_i = z_i + t_z * u_i$,    $z'_i = z'_i + t_z * u'_i$.
4. $X = [x_1, x_2, \ldots, x_{p_x}]$, $Z = [z_1, z_2, \ldots, z_{p_z}]$.
5. $X' = [x'_1, x'_2, \ldots, x'_{p_x}]$, $Z' = [z'_1, z'_2, \ldots, z'_{p_z}]$.
6. $U = [u_1, u_2, \ldots, u_{p_u}]$, $y = U\beta_u + \epsilon$ where $\epsilon \in \mathcal{R}^n$ distributed i.i.d. MVN$(0, \sigma^2 I_n)$.

There is sparsity in the solution since a subset of columns of $X$ and $Z$ are independent of the latent factors used to generate $y$. We use 10-fold CV to select the optimal values of hyperparameters. We compare the following methods: (1) separate $X$ and separate $Z$ on the labeled data: the standard lasso is applied on the separate data modalities of $X$ and $Z$ with 10-fold CV; (2) early fusion on the labeled data: the standard lasso is applied on the concatenated data modalities of $X$ and $Z$ with 10-fold CV (note that this is equivalent to cooperative learning with $\rho = 0$); (3) late fusion on the labeled data: separate lasso models are first fitted on $X$ and $Z$ independently with 10-fold CV, and the two resulting predictors are then combined through linear least squares for the final prediction; (4) cooperative learning on the labeled data; (5) semi-supervised cooperative learning on both the labeled and unlabeled data[3].

Overall, the simulation results can be summarized as follows:

- Semi-supervised cooperative learning performs the best in terms of test MSE across the range of SNR and correlation settings. It is most helpful when the data views are correlated and both contain signals, as shown in Fig. 2A.
- When there is no correlation between data views but each data view carries signals, semi-supervised cooperative learning still offers performance advantages as it utilizes the signals in both labeled and unlabled data, as shown in Fig. 2C.
- When the correlation between data views is higher, higher values of $\rho$ are more likely to be selected, as shown in Fig. 2B compared to Fig. 2A. In addition, cooperative learning-based methods tend to select more features.

---

[3] Traditional supervised learning models are not directly applicable to scenarios involving both labeled and unlabeled data.

## 3.2    Real Data Example

We applied semi-supervised cooperative learning to a real multiomics dataset of aging, collected from a cohort of 100 healthy individuals and individuals with prediabetes, as described in [28]. Proteomics and transcriptomics were measured on the cohort: the proteomics data contained measurements for 302 proteins and the transcriptomics data contained measurements for 8,556 genes. The goal of the analysis is to predict age using proteomics and transcriptomics data and uncover molecular signatures associated with the aging process.

We split the data set of 100 individuals into training and test sets of 75 and 25 individuals, respectively. We artificially masked the labels for half of the training samples to create a mix of labeled and unlabeled data. Both the proteomics and transcriptomics measurements were screened by their variance across the subjects. We averaged the expression levels for each individual across time points in the longitudinal study and predicted the corresponding age. We conducted the same set of experiments across 10 different random splits of the training and test sets.

**Table 1.** *Multiomics studies on aging.* The first two columns in the table show the mean and standard deviation (SD) of mean absolute error (MAE) on the test set across different splits of the training and test sets; the third and fourth columns show the MAE difference relative to early fusion. The methods include (1) separate proteomics: the standard lasso is applied on the proteomics data only; (2) separate transcriptomics: the standard lasso is applied on the transcriptomics data only; (3) early fusion: the standard lasso is applied on the concatenated data of proteomics and transcriptomics data; (4) late fusion: separate lasso models are first fit on proteomics and transcriptomics independently and the predictors are then combined through linear least squares; (5) cooperative learning; (6) semi-supervised cooperative learning.

| Methods | Test MAE | | Relative to Late Fusion | |
|---|---|---|---|---|
| | Mean | Std | Mean | Std |
| Separate Proteomics | 8.49 | 0.40 | −0.04 | 0.12 |
| Separate Transcriptomics | 8.44 | 0.35 | −0.08 | 0.20 |
| Early fusion | 8.52 | 0.32 | 0 | 0 |
| Late fusion | 8.53 | 0.29 | 0.01 | 0.13 |
| **Cooperative learning** | 8.16 | 0.40 | −0.37 | 0.16 |
| **Semi-supervised cooperative learning** | **7.85** | **0.47** | **−0.67** | **0.26** |

The results are shown in Table 1. The model fit on the transcriptomics data achieves lower test MAE than the one fit on the proteomics data. Early and late fusion hurt performance as compared to the model fit on only proteomics or transcriptomics. Cooperative learning outperforms both early and late fusion by encouraging the predictions to align with each other. Semi-supervised cooperative learning gives further performance gains by utilizing both the labeled and unlabeled data. Moreover, it selects important features not identified by the other methods for predicting age, including PDK1, MYSM1, ATP5A1, APOA4, MST, A2M, which have been previously demonstrated to be associated with the aging process [1,2,7,10,12,17,22,23].

## 4   Conclusion

We introduce semi-supervised cooperative learning for multiomics data fusion in the presence of both labeled and unlabeled data. By exploiting the shared underlying relationships across omics through an agreement penalty in both labeled and unlabeled data, our proposed approach demonstrates improved predictive accuracy on simulated studies and a real multiomics study of aging. The agreement penalty allows us to effectively incorporate the unlabeled samples in the learning process and leverage them to our advantage. To our knowledge, our work represents a pioneering effort in multi-omics data fusion that unlocks the untapped potential of unlabeled data, enabling us to harness the valuable information that would otherwise remain unused for the discovery of novel insights and enhanced predictive modeling of diagnostics and therapeutics.

## References

1. An, S., et al.: Inhibition of 3-phosphoinositide-dependent protein kinase 1 (pdk1) can revert cellular senescence in human dermal fibroblasts. Proc. Natl. Acad. Sci. **117**(49), 31535–31546 (2020)
2. Blacker, D., et al.: Alpha-2 macroglobulin is genetically associated with Alzheimer disease. Nat. Genet. **19**(4), 357–360 (1998)
3. Chabon, J.J., et al.: Integrating genomic features for non-invasive early lung cancer detection. Nature **580**(7802), 245–251 (2020)
4. Chaudhary, K., Poirion, O.B., Lu, L., Garmire, L.X.: Deep learning-based multiomics integration robustly predicts survival in liver cancer. Clin. Cancer Res. **24**(6), 1248–1259 (2018)
5. Chen, R.J., et al.: Pathomic fusion: an integrated framework for fusing histopathology and genomic features for cancer diagnosis and prognosis. IEEE Trans. Med. Imaging **41**(4), 757–770 (2022). https://doi.org/10.1109/TMI.2020.3021387
6. Chen, T., Kornblith, S., Norouzi, M., Hinton, G.: A simple framework for contrastive learning of visual representations. In: International Conference on Machine Learning, pp. 1597–1607. PMLR (2020)
7. Choi, S.Y., et al.: C9orf72-als/ftd-associated poly (GR) binds atp5a1 and compromises mitochondrial function in vivo. Nat. Neurosci. **22**(6), 851–862 (2019)
8. Ding, D.Y., Li, S., Narasimhan, B., Tibshirani, R.: Cooperative learning for multiview analysis. Proc. Natl. Acad. Sci. **119**(38), e2202113119 (2022)
9. Friedman, J., Hastie, T., Tibshirani, R.: Regularization paths for generalized linear models via coordinate descent. J. Stat. Softw. **33**, 1–22 (2010)
10. Garasto, S., et al.: The study of apoa1, apoc3 and apoa4 variability in healthy ageing people reveals another paradox in the oldest old subjects. Ann. Hum. Genet. **67**(1), 54–62 (2003)

11. Gentles, A.J., et al.: Integrating tumor and stromal gene expression signatures with clinical indices for survival stratification of early-stage non-small cell lung cancer. JNCI: J. Natl. Cancer Inst. **107**(10) (2015)
12. Goldberg, J., et al.: The mitochondrial ATP synthase is a shared drug target for aging and dementia. Aging Cell **17**(2), e12715 (2018)
13. Hao, Y., et al.: Integrated analysis of multimodal single-cell data. Cell **184**(13), 3573–3587 (2021)
14. Karczewski, K.J., Snyder, M.P.: Integrative omics for health and disease. Nat. Rev. Genet. **19**(5), 299 (2018)
15. Khosla, P., et al.: Supervised contrastive learning. In: Proceedings of the 34th Conference on Neural Information Processing Systems (2020)
16. Kristensen, V.N., Lingjærde, O.C., Russnes, H.G., Vollan, H.K.M., Frigessi, A., Børresen-Dale, A.L.: Principles and methods of integrative genomic analyses in cancer. Nat. Rev. Cancer **14**(5), 299–313 (2014)
17. Lee, J.K., et al.: MST1 functions as a key modulator of neurodegeneration in a mouse model of ALS. Proc. Natl. Acad. Sci. **110**(29), 12066–12071 (2013)
18. Ma, A., McDermaid, A., Xu, J., Chang, Y., Ma, Q.: Integrative methods and practical challenges for single-cell multi-omics. Trends Biotechnol. **38**(9), 1007–1022 (2020)
19. Perkins, B.A., et al.: Precision medicine screening using whole-genome sequencing and advanced imaging to identify disease risk in adults. Proc. Natl. Acad. Sci. **115**(14), 3686–3691 (2018)
20. Ritchie, M.D., Holzinger, E.R., Li, R., Pendergrass, S.A., Kim, D.: Methods of integrating data to uncover genotype-phenotype interactions. Nat. Rev. Genet. **16**(2), 85–97 (2015)
21. Robinson, D.R., et al.: Integrative clinical genomics of metastatic cancer. Nature **548**(7667), 297–303 (2017)
22. Shang, H., et al.: Role of MST1 in the regulation of autophagy and mitophagy: implications for aging-related diseases. J. Physiol. Biochem. 1–11 (2022)
23. Tian, M., et al.: MYSM1 suppresses cellular senescence and the aging process to prolong lifespan. Adv. Sci. **7**(22), 2001950 (2020)
24. Wu, L., et al.: An integrative multi-omics analysis to identify candidate DNA methylation biomarkers related to prostate cancer risk. Nat. Commun. **11**(1), 1–11 (2020)
25. Yang, P., Hwa Yang, Y., Zhou, B.B., Zomaya, A.Y.: A review of ensemble methods in bioinformatics. Curr. Bioinform. **5**(4), 296–308 (2010)
26. Yuan, Y., et al.: Assessing the clinical utility of cancer genomic and proteomic data across tumor types. Nat. Biotechnol. **32**(7), 644–652 (2014)
27. Zhao, J., et al.: Learning from longitudinal data in electronic health record and genetic data to improve cardiovascular event prediction. Sci. Rep. **9**(1), 1–10 (2019)
28. Zhou, W., et al.: Longitudinal multi-omics of host-microbe dynamics in prediabetes. Nature **569**(7758), 663–671 (2019)

# Exploiting Partial Common Information Microstructure for Multi-modal Brain Tumor Segmentation

Yongsheng Mei$^{(\boxtimes)}$ [ID], Guru Venkataramani [ID], and Tian Lan [ID]

The George Washington University, Washington DC 20052, USA
{ysmei,guruv,tlan}@gwu.edu

**Abstract.** Learning with multiple modalities is crucial for automated brain tumor segmentation from magnetic resonance imaging data. Explicitly optimizing the common information shared among all modalities (e.g., by maximizing the total correlation) has been shown to achieve better feature representations and thus enhance the segmentation performance. However, existing approaches are oblivious to partial common information shared by subsets of the modalities. In this paper, we show that identifying such partial common information can significantly boost the discriminative power of image segmentation models. In particular, we introduce a novel concept of partial common information mask (PCI-mask) to provide a fine-grained characterization of what partial common information is shared by which subsets of the modalities. By solving a masked correlation maximization and simultaneously learning an optimal PCI-mask, we identify the latent microstructure of partial common information and leverage it in a self-attention module to selectively weight different feature representations in multi-modal data. We implement our proposed framework on the standard U-Net. Our experimental results on the Multi-modal Brain Tumor Segmentation Challenge (BraTS) datasets outperform those of state-of-the-art segmentation baselines, with validation Dice similarity coefficients of 0.920, 0.897, 0.837 for the whole tumor, tumor core, and enhancing tumor on BraTS-2020.

**Keywords:** Multi-modal learning · Image segmentation · Maximal correlation optimization · Common information

## 1 Introduction

Brain tumor segmentation from magnetic resonance imaging (MRI) data is necessary for the diagnosis, monitoring, and treatment planning of the brain diseases. Since manual annotation by specialists is time-consuming and expensive, recently, automated segmentation approaches powered by deep-learning-based methods have become ever-increasingly prevailing in coping with various tumors in medical images. FCN [21], U-Net [34], and V-Net [27] are popular networks for medical image segmentation, to which many other optimization strategies have

© The Author(s), under exclusive license to Springer Nature Switzerland AG 2024
A. K. Maier et al. (Eds.): ML4MHD 2023, LNCS 14315, pp. 64–85, 2024.
https://doi.org/10.1007/978-3-031-47679-2_6

also been applied [5, 9, 17, 45]. The MRI data for segmentation usually has multiple modalities where each modality will convey different information and has its unique concentration. Due to this benefit, various approaches [15, 16, 32, 38, 40] for segmenting multi-modal MRI images regarding brain tumors have been proposed with improved results.

In practice, the multi-modal data allows the identification of common information shared by different modalities and from complementary views [12], thus achieving better representations by the resulting neural networks. From the information theory perspective, the most informative structure between modalities represents the feature representation of one modality that carries the maximum amount of information towards another one [11]. Efficiently leveraging common information among multiple modalities will uncover their latent relations and lead to superior performance.

To this end, we propose a novel framework that can leverage the partial common information microstructure of multiple modalities in brain tumor segmentation tasks. Specifically, we formulate an optimization problem where its objective, masked correlation, is defined as the sum of a series of correlation functions concerning the partial common information mask (PCI-mask). PCI-masks contain variable weights that can be assigned for different feature representations selectively. By solving the masked correlation maximization, we can obtain specific weights in PCI-masks and explicitly identify the hidden microstructure of partial common information in multi-modal data. In contrast to existing works [12, 13, 41] that employ a maximal correlation (e.g., Hirschfeld-Gebelein-Renyi (HGR) maximal correlation [33]) to find the maximally non-linear correlated feature representations of modalities, we adopt the PCI-mask to identify a fine-grained characterization of the latent partial common information shared by subsets of different modalities. Meanwhile, during learning, we optimize and update PCI-masks in an online and unsupervised fashion to allow them to dynamically reflect the partial common information microstructure among modalities.

Solving the mentioned optimization problem generates the PCI-mask illuminating the principal hidden partial common information microstructure in feature representations of multi-modal data, visualized by dark regions in Fig. 2. To thoroughly exploit such an informative microstructure, we design a self-attention module taking the PCI-masks and concatenated feature representation of each modality as inputs to obtain the attention feature representation carrying precise partial common information. This module will discriminate different types and structures of partial common information by selectively assigning different attention weights. Thus, utilizing PCI-masks and the self-attention mechanism make our segmentation algorithm more capable of avoiding treating different modalities as equal contributors in training or over-aggressively maximizing the total correlation of feature representations.

Following the theoretical analysis, we propose a new semantic brain tumor segmentation algorithm leveraging PCI-masks. The proposed solution also applies to many image segmentation tasks involving multi-modal data. The backbone of this design is the vanilla multi-modal U-Net, with which we integrate two new modules, masked maximal correlation (MMC) and masked self-attention (MSA), representing the PCI-mask optimization and self-attention mechanism, respectively. Besides, we adopt the standard cross-entropy segmentation loss and newly derived masked maximal correlation loss in the proposed method, where the latter guides both the learning of feature representations and the optimization of PCI-masks.

Our proposed solution is evaluated on the public brain tumor dataset, Multi-modal Brain Tumor Segmentation Challenge (BraTS) [26], containing fully annotated multi-modal brain tumor MRI images. We validate the effectiveness of our method through comparisons with advanced brain tumor segmentation baselines and perform ablations regarding the contributions of designed modules. In experiments, our proposed method consistently indicates improved empirical performance over the state-of-the-art baselines, with validation Dice similarity coefficient of 0.920, 0.897, 0.837 for the whole tumor, tumor core, and enhancing tumor on BraTS-2020, respectively.

The main contributions of our work are as follows:

- We introduce the novel PCI-mask and its online optimization to identify partial common information microstructures in multi-modal data during learning.
- We propose a U-Net-based framework utilizing PCI-masks and the self-attention mechanism to exploit the partial common information thoroughly.
- Experimental results of our design demonstrate its effectiveness in handling brain tumor segmentation tasks outperforming state-of-the-art baselines.

## 2   Related Works

### 2.1   Medical Image Segmentation Approaches

Image processing and related topics has demonstrated the importance in multiple areas [39,42]. As a complicated task, automated medical image segmentation plays a vital role in disease diagnosis and treatment planning. In the early age, segmentation systems rely on traditional methods such as object edge detection filters and mathematical algorithms [18,28], yet their heavy computational complexity hinders the development. Recently, deep-learning-based segmentation techniques achieved remarkable success regarding processing speed and accuracy and became popular for medical image segmentation. FCN [21] utilized the full convolution to handle pixel-wise prediction, becoming a milestone of medical image segmentation. Later-proposed U-Net [34] designed a symmetric encoder-decoder architecture with skip connections, where the encoding path captures context information and the decoding path ensures the accurate location. Due to the improved segmentation behavior of U-Net, numerous U-Net-based variances for brain tumor segmentation have been introduced, such as additional residual connections [9,14,17], densely connected layers [10,24], and extension with an extra decoder [29]. Besides, as the imitation of human perception, the attention mechanism can highlight useful information while suppressing the redundant remains. As shown in many existing works [32, 35, 43], attention structures or embedded attention modules can also effectively improve brain tumor segmentation performance. In this paper, we use U-Net as the backbone integrated with newly designed modules to thoroughly leverage partial common information microstructure among modalities often overlooked in segmentation.

### 2.2 HGR Correlation in Multi-modal Learning

The computation of the maximal correlation has been adopted in many multi-modal learning practices for feature extraction. As a generalization from Pearson's correlation [31], the HGR maximal correlation is prevailing for its legitimacy as a measure of dependency. In the view of information theory, the HGR transformation carries the maximum amount of information of a specific modality to another and vice versa. For instance, [8] shows that maximizing the HGR maximal correlation allows determining the nonlinear transformation of two maximally correlated variables. Soft-HGR loss is introduced in [37] as the development of standard HGR maximal correlation to extract the most informative features from different modalities. These works and other variants [12, 13, 41] validate the effectiveness of maximal correlation methods in extracting features by conducting experiments on simple datasets, such as CIFAR-10 [20]. Additionally, [23, 44] adopt the Soft-HGR loss for the other multi-modal learning task, which is emotion recognition. In this work, we further develop the Soft-HGR technique to extract optimal partial informative feature representations through the PCI-mask and leverage them for brain tumor segmentation.

## 3  Background

### 3.1  Brain Tumor Segmentation

Brain tumors refer to the abnormal and uncontrolled multiplication of pathological cells growing in or around the human brain tissue. We can categorize brain tumors into primary and secondary tumor types [7] based on their different origins. For primary ones, the abnormal growth of cells initiates inside the brain, whereas secondary tumors' cancerous cells metastasize into the brain from other body organs such as lungs and kidneys. The most common malignant primary brain tumors are gliomas, arising from brain glial cells, which can either be fast-growing high-grade gliomas (HGG) or slow-growing low-grade gliomas (LGG) [22]. Magnetic resonance imaging (MRI) is a standard noninvasive imaging technique that can display detailed images of the brain and soft tissue contrast without latent injury and skull artifacts, which is adopted in many different tasks [2, 3]. In usual practices, complimentary MRI modalities are available: T1-weighted (T1), T2-weighted (T2), T1-weighted with contrast agent (T1c), and fluid attenuation inversion recovery (FLAIR) [1], which emphasize different tissue properties and areas of tumor spread. To support clinical application and scientific research, brain tumor segmentation over multi-modal MRI data has become an essential task in medical image processing [6].

## 3.2 HGR Maximal Correlation

The HGR maximal correlation was originally defined on a single feature, while we can easily extend it to scenarios with multiple features involved. Considering a dataset with $k$ modalities, we define the multi-model observations as $k$-tuples, i.e., $(X_1, \cdots, X_k)$. For the $i$-th modality, we use a transformation function $\boldsymbol{f}_i(X_i) = [f_1^{(i)}(X_i), \ldots, f_m^{(i)}(X_i)]^T$ to compute its $m$-dimensional feature representation. Based on given definitions, the HGR maximal correlation is defined as follows:

$$\rho(X_i, X_j) = \sup_{\substack{X_i, X_j \in \mathbb{R}^k \\ \mathbb{E}[f_i] = \mathbb{E}[f_j] = 0 \\ \boldsymbol{\Sigma}_{f_i} = \boldsymbol{\Sigma}_{f_j} = \mathbf{I}}} \mathbb{E}[\boldsymbol{f}_i^T(X_i)\boldsymbol{f}_j(X_j)],$$

where $i$ and $j$ ranges from 1 to $k$, and $\boldsymbol{\Sigma}$ denotes the covariance of the feature representation. The supremum is taken over all sets of Borel measurable functions with zero-mean and identity covariance. Since finding the HGR maximal correlation will lead us to locate the informative non-linear transformations of feature representations $\boldsymbol{f}_i$ and $\boldsymbol{f}_j$ from different modalities, it becomes useful to extract features with more common information from multi-modal data.

## 3.3 Soft-HGR

Compared to the traditional HGR maximal correlation method, Soft-HGR adopts a low-rank approximation, making it more suitable for high-dimensional data. Maximizing a Soft-HGR objective has been shown to extract hidden common information features among multiple modalities more efficiently [37]. The optimization problem to maximize the multi-modal Soft-HGR maximal correlation is described as follows:

$$\max_{f_1, \ldots, f_k} \sum_{\substack{i,j=1 \\ i \neq j}}^{k} L(\boldsymbol{f}_i(X_i), \boldsymbol{f}_j(X_j)) \tag{1}$$

$$\text{s.t.} \quad X_i, X_j \in \mathbb{R}^k, \mathbb{E}[\boldsymbol{f}_i(X_i)] = \mathbb{E}[\boldsymbol{f}_j(X_j)] = \mathbf{0},$$

where, given $i$ and $j$ ranging from 1 to $k$, feature representations $\boldsymbol{f}_i$ and $\boldsymbol{f}_j$ should satisfy zero-mean condition, and the function of the optimization objective in Eq. (1) is:

$$L(\boldsymbol{f}_i, \boldsymbol{f}_j) \stackrel{\text{def}}{=} \mathbb{E}[\boldsymbol{f}_i^T(X_i)\boldsymbol{f}_j(X_j)] - \frac{1}{2}\text{tr}(\boldsymbol{\Sigma}_{f_i(X_i)}\boldsymbol{\Sigma}_{f_j(X_j)}), \tag{2}$$

where $\text{tr}(\cdot)$ denotes the trace of its matrix argument and $\boldsymbol{\Sigma}$ is the covariance. We note that Eq. (2) contains two inner products: the first term is between feature representations representing the objective of the HGR maximal correlation; the second term is between their covariance, which is the proposed soft regularizer to replace the whitening constraints.

# 4  Identifying Partial Common Information

## 4.1  Masked Correlation Maximization

We first introduce a special mask to the standard Soft-HGR optimization problem. The introduced mask can selectively assign variable weights for feature representations and aims to identify the latent partial common information microstructure at specific dimensions of feature representations implied by higher mask weights. Such high weights add importance and compel the common information to concentrate on a subset of feature representations from different modalities when computing the maximal correlation. Thus, by applying the mask, we can differentiate critical partial common information from its trivial counterpart in feature representations effectively and precisely.

Based on the function $L(\boldsymbol{f}_i, \boldsymbol{f}_j)$ in Eq. (2), we apply a selective mask vector $\boldsymbol{s}$ to input feature representations $\boldsymbol{f}_i(X_i)$ and $\boldsymbol{f}_j(X_j)$ by computing their element-wise products. The vector $\boldsymbol{s}$ shares the same dimension $m$ with feature representations, such that $\boldsymbol{s} = [s_1, \cdots, s_m]^{\mathrm{T}}$. We restrict the value of mask weights to $[0,1]$ with higher weights representing the more concentration to feature representations' dimensions with more latent partial common information. We also consider a constraint on the sum of mask weights, i.e., $\mathbf{1}^{\mathrm{T}}\boldsymbol{s} \leq c$ with a predefined constant $c > 0$ in order to let the common information mask focus on at most $c$ dimensions with the most valuable common information in feature representations. The reformatted maximal correlation optimization problem in Eq. (1) with function $L(\boldsymbol{f}_i, \boldsymbol{f}_j)$ becomes:

$$\max_{\boldsymbol{f}_1, \ldots, \boldsymbol{f}_k} \sum_{\substack{i,j=1 \\ i \neq j}}^{k} \bar{L}(\boldsymbol{s}_{ij} \odot \boldsymbol{f}_i, \boldsymbol{s}_{ij} \odot \boldsymbol{f}_j), \tag{3}$$

where $\odot$ denotes the element-wise product. We can notice that the weights of the selective mask vector are directly applied to the input feature representations. When solving the optimization problem in Eq. (3), this product will only emphasize the feature dimensions consisting of latent common information microstructure among feature representations from different modalities.

The selective mask vectors $\boldsymbol{s}_{ij}$ in Eq. (3) need to be optimized to explicitly identify the microstructure between feature representations. However, it is inefficient to directly solve the optimization problem in Eq. (3) with selective mask vectors. To address this issue, we consider an equivalent optimization with respect to a partial common information mask (PCI-mask) $\boldsymbol{\Lambda}$ defined as follows:

**Definition 1 (Partial common information mask).** *We define PCI-mask as a $m \times m$ diagonal matrix $\mathrm{diag}(\lambda_1, \ldots, \lambda_i)$ with diagonal values denoted by $\lambda_i$, where $i = 1, \ldots, m$.*

After giving the definition of PCI-mask, we provide the masked maximal correlation for identifying optimal common information through a new optimization problem with necessary constraints.

**Theorem 1 (Masked maximal correlation).** *The optimization of maximal correlation with respect to selective mask vectors $s$ in Eq. (3) is equivalent to the following optimization over PCI-mask $\boldsymbol{\Lambda}$ with zero-mean feature representation $\boldsymbol{f}_i(X_i)$ of $k$ modalities:*

$$\max_{\boldsymbol{f}_1,\dots,\boldsymbol{f}_k} \sum_{\substack{i,j=1 \\ i\neq j}}^{k} \tilde{L}(\boldsymbol{f}_i, \boldsymbol{f}_j, \boldsymbol{\Lambda}_{ij}), \tag{4a}$$

*where the function $\tilde{L}(\boldsymbol{f}_i, \boldsymbol{f}_j, \boldsymbol{\Lambda}_{ij})$ is given by:*

$$\tilde{L}(\boldsymbol{f}_i, \boldsymbol{f}_j, \boldsymbol{\Lambda}_{ij}) \stackrel{\text{def}}{=} \mathbb{E}\left[\boldsymbol{f}_i^{\mathrm{T}}(X_i)\boldsymbol{\Lambda}_{ij}\boldsymbol{f}_j(X_j)\right] - \frac{1}{2}\mathrm{tr}\left(\boldsymbol{\Sigma}_{\boldsymbol{f}_i(X_i)}\boldsymbol{\Lambda}_{ij}\boldsymbol{\Sigma}_{\boldsymbol{f}_j(X_j)}\boldsymbol{\Lambda}_{ij}\right), \tag{4b}$$

*and the PCI-mask $\boldsymbol{\Lambda}$ satisfies the following conditions:*

*1) Range constraint: The diagonal values of $\boldsymbol{\Lambda}$ falls in $0 \le \lambda_i \le 1$;*
*2) Sum constraint: The sum of diagonal values are bounded: $\sum_{i=1}^{m} \lambda_i \le c$.*

*Proof.* See Appendix A.

The PCI-mask in Eq. (4b) captures the precise location of partial common information between feature representations of different modalities and allows efficient maximal correlation calculation in Eq. (4a). However, as learned feature representations will vary during the training process, a static PCI-mask will be insufficient for obtaining the latent microstructure. Therefore, to synchronize with learned feature representations, we optimize the PCI-mask in an unsupervised manner for each learning step.

### 4.2    Learning Microstructure via PCI-Mask Update

To optimize PCI-mask under two constraints mentioned in Theorem 1, we adopt the projected gradient descent (PGD) method. PGD is a standard approach to solve the constrained optimization problem, allowing updating the PCI-mask in an unsupervised and online fashion during the learning process.

Optimizing the PCI-mask with PGD requires two key steps: (1) selecting an initial starting point within the constraint set and (2) iteratively updating the gradient and projecting it on to the feasibility set. In accordance to both range and sum constraints in Theorem 1, we define a feasibility set as $\mathcal{Q} = \{\boldsymbol{\Lambda}|\boldsymbol{\Lambda}_{i,i} \in [0,1]\ \forall i,\ \mathbf{1}^{\mathrm{T}}\boldsymbol{\Lambda}\mathbf{1} \le c\}$. Then, we iteratively compute the gradient descent from an initial PCI-mask $\boldsymbol{\Lambda}_0$ ($n = 0$) and project the updated PCI-mask on to $\mathcal{Q}$:

$$\boldsymbol{\Lambda}_{n+1} = P_{\mathcal{Q}}(\boldsymbol{\Lambda}_n - \alpha_n \frac{\partial \tilde{L}}{\partial \boldsymbol{\Lambda}_n}), \tag{5}$$

where $n$ denotes the current step, $P_{\mathcal{Q}}(\cdot)$ represents the projection operator, and $\alpha_n \ge 0$ is the step size.

We first introduce the following lemma as the key ingredient for deriving the gradient descent.

**Lemma 1 (Mask gradient).** *For $k$ modalities, the gradient with respect to PCI-mask is given by:*

$$\frac{\partial \tilde{L}}{\partial \mathbf{\Lambda}} = \sum_{\substack{i,j=1 \\ i \neq j}}^{k} \frac{\partial \tilde{L}(\mathbf{f}_i, \mathbf{f}_j, \mathbf{\Lambda}_{ij})}{\partial \mathbf{\Lambda}_{ij}},$$

*where the partial derivation with respect to $\mathbf{\Lambda}_{ij}$ is:*

$$\frac{\partial \tilde{L}(\mathbf{f}_i, \mathbf{f}_j, \mathbf{\Lambda}_{ij})}{\partial \mathbf{\Lambda}_{ij}} = \mathbb{E}\left[\mathbf{f}_j(X_j)\mathbf{f}_i^{\mathrm{T}}(X_i)\right] - \frac{1}{2}\left[\left(\mathbf{\Sigma}_{\mathbf{f}_i(X_i)}\mathbf{\Lambda}_{ij}\mathbf{\Sigma}_{\mathbf{f}_j(X_j)}\right)^{\mathrm{T}} + \left(\mathbf{\Sigma}_{\mathbf{f}_j(X_j)}\mathbf{\Lambda}_{ij}\mathbf{\Sigma}_{\mathbf{f}_i(X_i)}\right)^{\mathrm{T}}\right].$$

*Proof.* See Appendix B.

Lemma 1 provides the computational result for Eq. (5). Since the PCI-mask is updated in a unsupervised manner, we will terminate the gradient descent process when confirming the satisfaction of a stopping condition, such as the difference between the current gradient and a predefined threshold being smaller than a tolerable error. Besides, as shown in Eq. (5), we apply the projection to descended gradient, and this projection is also an optimization problem. More specifically, given a point $\bar{\mathbf{\Lambda}} = \mathbf{\Lambda}_n - \alpha_n(\partial \tilde{L}/\partial \mathbf{\Lambda}_n)$, $P_{\mathcal{Q}}$ will find another feasible point $\mathbf{\Lambda}_{n+1} \in \mathcal{Q}$ with the minimum Euclidean distance to $\bar{\mathbf{\Lambda}}$, which is:

$$P_{\mathcal{Q}}(\bar{\mathbf{\Lambda}}) = \arg\min_{\mathbf{\Lambda}_{n+1}} \frac{1}{2}\|\mathbf{\Lambda}_{n+1} - \bar{\mathbf{\Lambda}}\|_2^2. \tag{6}$$

Equation (6) indicates the projection mechanism by selecting a valid candidate with the shortest distance to the current point at step $n$ within the defined feasibility set. Combining this procedure with the gradient descent, the constraints in Theorem 1 will always hold for the updated PCI-mask during unsupervised optimization. Therefore, the partial common information microstructure can be effectively identified from feature representations through the optimized PCI-mask, in which the weights will be increased for dimensions exhibiting higher partial common information.

## 5    System Design

### 5.1    Model Learning

The multi-modal image segmentation task requires well-learned feature representations and common information microstructure to improve performance. Therefore, we consider the segmentation and partial common information microstructure exploitation simultaneously by defining the total loss function $\mathcal{L}_{tot}$ of our model as follows:

$$\mathcal{L}_{tot} = \theta\mathcal{L}_{corr} + \mathcal{L}_{ce}, \tag{7}$$

where $\mathcal{L}_{corr}$ is the masked maximal correlation loss, and $\mathcal{L}_{ce}$ denotes the standard cross-entropy segmentation loss. The parameter $\theta$ is the weighting factor for correlation loss to keep both loss functions proportionally in a similar scale.

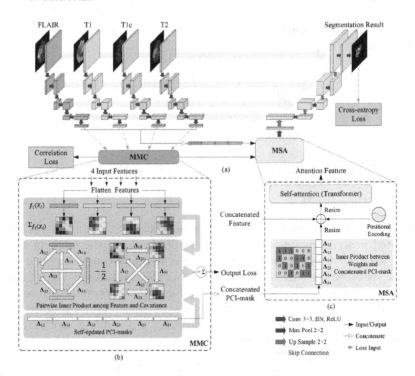

**Fig. 1.** The architecture overview (a) of the designed system. Beyond the U-Net backbone, the system contains two newly designed modules: Masked Maximal Correlation (MMC) module (b) and Masked Self-Attention (MSA) module (c). We use the total loss consisting of weighted masked maximum correlation loss and cross-entropy segmentation loss to train the model.

Based on Theorem 1, we define the masked maximal correlation loss as the negative of the function in Eq. (4b), such that $\mathcal{L}_{corr} = -\tilde{L}$. It changes the maximizing correlation problem to minimizing the correlation loss, and both are equivalent regarding using the partial common information from multi-modal data. We provide the procedure of masked maximal correlation loss computation in Appendix C.1. Besides, Algorithm 1 summarizes the detailed procedure of realizing unsupervised optimization of PCI-mask in Eq. (5), where we design a truncation function to project all the values of the PCI-mask into the space $[0, 1]$ to satisfy the range constraint. Furthermore, we leverage the bisection search to adjust element values in PCI-mask to guarantee that their sum remains no more than a predefined threshold during optimization as described by sum constraint.

For the segmentation loss in Eq. (7), we adopt the standard cross-entropy loss to guide the learning process. Finally, the weighted summation of two losses will participate in the backward propagation of the network.

---

**Algorithm 1.** Unsupervised optimization of PCI-mask using PGD

---

**Input**: Correlation loss $\mathcal{L}_{corr}$, PCI-mask $\mathbf{\Lambda}$
**Parameter**: Size of PCI-mask $m$, Step size $\alpha$, sum threshold $c$, lower and upper guesses $b_1, b_2$, tolerable error $e$
**Output**: Updated PCI-mask $\mathbf{\Lambda}'$

1: Compute the gradient descent:
    $\tilde{\mathbf{\Lambda}} \leftarrow \mathbf{\Lambda} - \alpha(\partial \mathcal{L}_{corr}/\partial \mathbf{\Lambda})$
2: Computing truncated PCI-mask:
    $\bar{\mathbf{\Lambda}} \leftarrow \text{truncate}(\tilde{\mathbf{\Lambda}})$
3: Comparing the sum with predefined threshold:
4: **if** $\sum_{i=1}^{n} \bar{\lambda}_i > c$ **then**
5:     Using bisection search: adjust $\bar{\lambda}_i$ value in $\bar{\mathbf{\Lambda}}$
6:     **while** $|\sum_{i=1}^{n} \bar{\lambda}_i - c| > e$ **do**
7:         $r \leftarrow (b_1 + b_2)/2$
8:         **for** $i = 1 : m$ **do**
9:             $\bar{\lambda}_i \leftarrow \text{truncate}(\bar{\lambda}_i - r)$
10:        **end for**
11:       **if** $\sum_{i=1}^{n} \bar{\lambda}_i > c$ **then**
12:          $b_1 \leftarrow r$
13:       **else**
14:          $b_2 \leftarrow r$
15:       **end if**
16:     **end while**
17: **end if**
18: **return** $\mathbf{\Lambda}' \leftarrow \bar{\mathbf{\Lambda}}$

*Routine* truncate($\cdot$). See Appendix C.2.

---

## 5.2   Model Design

Figure 1 shows the whole system architecture of our design. Our model adopts the vanilla multi-modal U-Net as the main backbone, including encoding and decoding paths. The encoding path learns high-level feature representations from input data, while the decoding path up-samples the feature representations to generate pixel-wise segmentation results. Furthermore, the model concatenates the feature representations from the encoding to the decoding path by leveraging the skip connection to retain more information. In Fig. 1 (a), each convolution block contains a $3 \times 3$ convolution layer, followed by a batch normalization layer and a ReLU. Besides, the $2 \times 2$ max-pooling layer is adopted to downsample the feature representations. We calculate the masked maximal correlation loss by using the high-level feature representation at the end of each encoding path and compute the cross-entropy segmentation loss at the end of the decoding path.

    To explicitly identify and exploit partial common information during learning, we design two independent modules in Fig. 1 (a) to process learned high-level feature representations: the masked maximal correlation (MMC) and masked self-attention (MSA) modules. The details of the MMC module are shown in Fig. 1 (b). We first calculate the covariance matrices based on flattened input feature representations. Then, we use the PCI-masks to compute the inner prod-

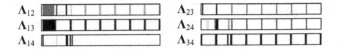

**Fig. 2.** Visualization of PCI-masks in gray-scale heat maps, where dark areas highlight the partial common information microstructure. Subscripts of PCI-mask $\Lambda$ ranging from 1 to 4 denote modalities FLAIR, T1, T1c, and T2, respectively.

uct among feature representations and covariance matrices, thereby getting the masked maximal correlation loss. The PCI-masks can reflect latent partial common information microstructures, as illustrated by the visualization in Fig. 2 where we show the PCI-masks in gray-scale heat maps. We can observe similar partial common information patterns (represented by dark areas) among different modalities that facilitate the segmentation. Meanwhile, the concatenation of all PCI-masks will be cached and passed into the next module.

We also apply the self-attention mechanism mentioned in [30,32,35] to the MSA module placed between the encoding and decoding paths given in Fig. 1 (c). We feed the MSA module with the partial common information microstructure stored in the PCI-mask and concatenated feature representation to predict the segmentation results accurately. As shown in Fig. 1 (c), we apply an additional 4 × 6 attention weight matrix to the concatenated PCI-mask. This weight matrix is designed to search for the best combination of all PCI-masks that can select the common information most relevant to one modality. After that, the chosen combination will become one of the inputs of the self-attention module core. We will extract an attention feature representation as the final output of the MSA module.

## 6    Experiments

In this section, we provided experimental results on BraTS-2020 datasets by comparing our model with state-of-the-art baselines, reporting in several metrics. We also visualized and analyze the PCI-masks and the segmentation results of our design. Additionally, we investigated the impact of the weighting factor and used several ablations to discuss the contribution of MMC and MSA modules shown in Fig. 1. More results using an older BraTS dataset and implementation details are provided in Appendix D. Code has been made available at: https://github.com/ysmei97/multimodal_pci_mask.

### 6.1    Datasets

The BraTS-2020 training dataset consists of 369 multi-contrast MRI scans, where 293 have been acquired from HGG and 76 from LGG. All the multi-modality scans contain four modalities: FLAIR, T1, T1c, and T2. Each of these modalities captures different brain tumor sub-regions, including the necrotic and non-enhancing tumor core (NCR/NET) with label 1, peritumoral edema (ED) with label 2, and GD-enhancing tumor (ET) with label 4.

**Table 1.** Segmentation result comparisons between our framework and other baselines on the best single model.

| Baselines | DSC | | | Sensitivity | | | Specificity | | | PPV | | |
|---|---|---|---|---|---|---|---|---|---|---|---|---|
| | ET | WT | TC | ET | WT | TC | ET | WT | TC | ET | WT | TC |
| Vanilla U-Net | 0.822 | 0.883 | 0.867 | 0.816 | 0.880 | 0.831 | 0.998 | 0.998 | 0.999 | 0.856 | 0.909 | 0.842 |
| Modality-Pairing Net | 0.833 | 0.912 | 0.869 | **0.872** | 0.895 | 0.866 | **1.000** | **0.999** | 0.999 | 0.871 | 0.934 | 0.892 |
| nnU-Net | 0.818 | 0.911 | 0.871 | 0.843 | 0.864 | 0.853 | 0.999 | 0.998 | **1.000** | 0.885 | 0.942 | 0.893 |
| CI-Autoencoder | 0.774 | 0.871 | 0.840 | 0.780 | 0.844 | 0.792 | 0.998 | **0.999** | 0.999 | 0.892 | 0.921 | 0.885 |
| U-Net Transformer | 0.807 | 0.899 | 0.873 | 0.765 | 0.861 | 0.815 | 0.999 | **0.999** | **1.000** | 0.900 | 0.934 | 0.895 |
| Ours | **0.837** | **0.920** | **0.897** | 0.861 | **0.898** | **0.877** | **1.000** | **0.999** | **1.000** | **0.908** | **0.952** | **0.898** |

## 6.2   Data Preprocessing and Environmental Setup

The data are the 3D MRI images with the size of $155 \times 240 \times 240$. Due to their large size, we utilize slice-wise 2D segmentation to 3D biomedical data [4]. Therefore, all input MRI images are divided into 115 slices with the size of $240 \times 240$, which will be further normalized between 0 and 1. Then, we feed the processed images into our model and start training.

We adopt the grid search to determine the weighting factor in Eq. (7). The optimal value of $\theta$ is 0.003. We set the learning rate of the model to 0.0001 and the batch size to 32. The PCI-masks are randomly initialized. When optimizing the PCI-mask, step size $\alpha$ is set to 2, and tolerable error $e$ is set to 0.01 of the sum threshold. We enable the Adam optimizer [19] to train the model and set the maximum number of training epochs as 200. The designed framework is trained in an end-to-end manner.

## 6.3   Evaluation Metrics

We report our evaluation results in four metrics: Dice similarity coefficient (DSC), Sensitivity, Specificity, and positive predicted value (PPV). DSC measures volumetric overlap between segmentation results and annotations. Sensitivity and Specificity determine potential over/under-segmentations, where Sensitivity shows the percentage of correctly identified positive instances out of ground truth, while Specificity computes the proportion of correctly identified actual negatives. Besides, PPV calculates the probability of true positive instances out of positive results.

## 6.4   Main Results

Since BraTS evaluates segmentation using the partially overlapping whole tumor (WT), tumor core (TC), and enhancing tumor (ET) regions [26], optimizing these regions instead of the provided labels is beneficial for performance [17,36]. We train and validate our framework using five-fold cross-validation in a random split fashion on the training set. Then, we compare the results with original or

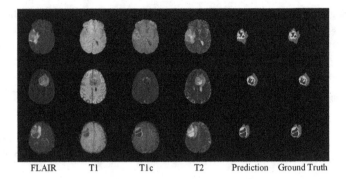

FLAIR        T1        T1c        T2        Prediction    Ground Truth

**Fig. 3.** Visualization of segmentation results. From left to right, we show axial slice of MRI images in four modalities, predicted segmentation, and ground truth. Labels include ED (cyan), ET (yellow), and NCR/NET (blue) for prediction and ground truth. (Color figure online)

**Table 2.** Searching the optimal weighting factor reporting DSC and sensitivity on whole tumor.

| Weight $\theta$ | 0.005 | 0.004 | **0.003** | 0.002 | 0.001 |
|---|---|---|---|---|---|
| DSC | 0.878 | 0.898 | **0.920** | 0.881 | 0.879 |
| Sensitivity | 0.854 | 0.886 | **0.898** | 0.883 | 0.864 |

reproduced results of advanced baselines, including vanilla U-Net [34], Modality-Pairing Network [38], nnU-Net [15], and U-Net Transformer [32]. The Modality-Pairing Network adopts a series of layer connections to capture complex relationships among modalities. Besides, nnU-Net is a robust and self-adapting extension to vanilla U-Net, setting many new state-of-the-art results. U-Net Transformer uses the U-Net with self-attention and cross-attention mechanisms embedded. Additionally, to demonstrate the effectiveness of optimized masked maximal correlation, we adapt the common information autoencoder (CI-Autoencoder) from [23] to our experimental setting and compute two pairwise correlations. Specifically, we create two static PCI-masks initialized as identity matrices and assign them to modality pairs FLAIR, T2, and T1, T1c.

We report the comparison results with other baselines in Table 1, where our proposed model achieves the best result. For instance, regarding DSC on WT, our method outperforms the vanilla U-Net by 3.7%. Also, our proposed method achieves higher scores concerning tumor regions of most other metrics. The results indicate that the exploitation of partial common information microstructure among modalities via PCI-masks can effectively improve segmentation performance. Moreover, we provide examples of segmentation results of our proposed design in Fig. 3. As can be seen, the segmentation results are sensibly identical to ground truth with accurate boundaries and some minor tumor areas identified.

**Table 3.** Ablations reporting DSC and sensitivity on whole tumor.

| Ablation | DSC | Sensitivity |
|----------|-----|-------------|
| 1: Soft-HGR | 0.882 | 0.871 |
| 2: MMC | 0.909 | 0.880 |
| 3: MSA | 0.899 | 0.861 |
| **4: MMC+MSA** | **0.920** | **0.898** |

As one of our main contributions, we visualize the PCI-masks to demonstrate captured partial common information microstructure and amount of partial common information varying between different feature representations and modalities. Due to the large dimension of the PCI-mask, we provide the first 128 diagonal element values of each PCI-mask in gray-scale heat maps in Fig. 2. The darker region represents higher weights, i.e., places with more partial common information. Given $\Lambda_{14}$ and $\Lambda_{34}$ in the figure, although we usually employ modalities FLAIR and T2 to extract features of the whole tumor, modality T1c still shares the microstructure with T2 that can assist identifying the whole tumor, told from their similar heat map patterns.

To investigate the impact of the weighting factor on the performance, we use grid search to search the optimal weight $\theta$ in Eq. (7). We show the results in Table 2 on BraTS-2020, where the best practice is $\theta = 0.003$. Since the value of correlation loss is much larger than the cross-entropy loss, we need to project both loss functions onto a similar scale to allow them to guide the learning process collaboratively. In the table, we can notice an apparent trend indicating a local optimum.

### 6.5  Ablation Experiments

We run several ablations to analyze our design. Results are shown in Table 3, where experiment 4 is our best practice.

**Static PCI-Mask vs. Optimized PCI-Mask:** The first ablation computes maximal correlations over all modalities, which is equivalent to assigning multiple static PCI-masks of identity matrices for every two modalities. Results in Table 3 show that the model benefits from self-optimized PCI-masks when comparing experiments 1 and 2 or experiments 3 and 4.

**Self-attention:** Comparing experiments 2 and 4 in Table 3, adding the MSA module improves the DSC by 1.1% and sensitivity score by 1.8%. This comparison demonstrates that applying the self-attention module to concentrate on the extracted common information allows better learning.

## 7  Conclusion

This paper proposes a novel method to exploit the partial common information microstructure for brain tumor segmentation. By solving a masked correlation maximization and simultaneously learning an optimal PCI-mask, we can identify and utilize the latent microstructure to selectively weight feature representations of different modalities. Our experimental results on BraTS-2020 show the validation DSC of 0.920, 0.897, 0.837 for the whole tumor, tumor core, and enhancing tumor, demonstrating superior segmentation performance over other baselines. We will extend the proposed method to more implementations in the future.

## A    Proof of Theorem 1

To begin with, we rewrite the covariance $\Sigma_{f_i(X_i)}$ and $\Sigma_{f_j(X_j)}$ by leveraging expectations of feature representations to get the unbiased estimators of the covariance matrices. The unbiased estimators of the covariance matrices are as follows:

$$\Sigma_{f_i(X_i)} = \mathbb{E}\left[f_i(X_i)f_i^{\mathrm{T}}(X_i)\right],$$
$$\Sigma_{f_j(X_j)} = \mathbb{E}\left[f_j(X_j)f_j^{\mathrm{T}}(X_j)\right].$$

Based on optimization problem (3), we apply the selective mask vector $s$ to input feature representations by leveraging the element-wise product. Per property that The element-wise product of two vectors is the same as the matrix multiplication of one vector by the corresponding diagonal matrix of the other vector, we have:

$$s \odot f = D_s f,$$

where $D_s$ represents the diagonal matrix with the same diagonal elements as the vector $s$.

The transpose of the diagonal matrix equals to itself. Therefore, the function $\bar{L}$ in (3) is now given by:

$$\bar{L}(s \odot f_i, s \odot f_j)$$
$$= \mathbb{E}\left[f_i^{\mathrm{T}}(X_i)D_s D_s f_j(X_j)\right] \tag{8a}$$
$$+ (\mathbb{E}\left[D_s f_i(X_i)\right])^{\mathrm{T}} \mathbb{E}\left[D_s f_j(X_j)\right] \tag{8b}$$
$$- \frac{1}{2}\mathrm{tr}\left\{\mathbb{E}\left[D_s f_i(X_i)f_i^{\mathrm{T}}(X_i)D_s\right] \mathbb{E}\left[D_s f_j(X_j)f_j^{\mathrm{T}}(X_j)D_s\right]\right\}. \tag{8c}$$

Considering that the input in Eq. (8a) subjects to zero-mean: $\mathbb{E}[f_i(X_i)] = 0$ for $i = 1, 2, \ldots, k$, the term (8b) becomes:

$$(\mathbb{E}\left[D_s f_i(X_i)\right])^{\mathrm{T}} \mathbb{E}\left[D_s f_j(X_j)\right] = 0.$$

Thus, (8b) can be omitted as it equals to 0. Using the property of matrix trace, the third term (8c) can be turned into:

$$- \frac{1}{2}\mathrm{tr}\left\{\mathbb{E}\left[D_s f_i(X_i)f_i^{\mathrm{T}}(X_i)D_s\right] \cdot \mathbb{E}\left[D_s f_j(X_j)f_j^{\mathrm{T}}(X_j)D_s\right]\right\}$$
$$= - \frac{1}{2}\mathrm{tr}\left\{\mathbb{E}\left[f_i(X_i)f_i^{\mathrm{T}}(X_i)\right] D_s D_s \cdot \mathbb{E}\left[f_j(X_j)f_j^{\mathrm{T}}(X_j)\right] D_s D_s\right\},$$

where the multiplication of two diagonal matrix $D_s$ is also a diagonal matrix with dimension of $m \times m$. Therefore, we define $\mathbf{\Lambda}$ as a diagonal matrix satisfying:

$$\mathbf{\Lambda} = D_s^2.$$

The constraints of the vector $\boldsymbol{s}$ are still applicable to $\mathbf{\Lambda}$. Using $\mathbf{\Lambda}$ to replace multiplications in terms (8a) and (8c), we have the equivalent function to (9a):

$$\tilde{L}(\boldsymbol{f}_i, \boldsymbol{f}_j, \mathbf{\Lambda}_{ij})$$

$$= \mathbb{E}\left[\boldsymbol{f}_i^{\mathrm{T}}(X_i)\mathbf{\Lambda}_{ij}\boldsymbol{f}_j(X_j)\right] \tag{9a}$$

$$- \frac{1}{2}\mathrm{tr}\left\{\mathbb{E}\left[\boldsymbol{f}_i(X_i)\boldsymbol{f}_i^{\mathrm{T}}(X_i)\right]\mathbf{\Lambda}_{ij}\mathbb{E}\left[\boldsymbol{f}_j(X_j)\boldsymbol{f}_j^{\mathrm{T}}(X_j)\right]\mathbf{\Lambda}_{ij}\right\}. \tag{9b}$$

# B Proof of Lemma 1

Given function $f$ with respect to matrix $X$, we can connect the matrix derivative with the total differential $df$ by:

$$df = \sum_{i=1}^{m}\sum_{j=1}^{n}\frac{\partial f}{\partial X_{i,j}}dX_{i,j} = \mathrm{tr}\left(\frac{\partial f^{\mathrm{T}}}{\partial X}dX\right). \tag{10}$$

Note that Eq. (10) still holds if the matrix $X$ is degraded to a vector $\boldsymbol{x}$.

The gradient computation in Lemma 1 is equivalent to computing the partial derivative regarding $\mathbf{\Lambda}_{ij}$ in Eq. (9a). To start with, we compute the total differential of first term (9a) as follows:

$$d\,\mathbb{E}\left[\boldsymbol{f}_i^{\mathrm{T}}(X_i)\mathbf{\Lambda}_{ij}\boldsymbol{f}_j(X_j)\right]$$

$$= \mathbb{E}\left[\boldsymbol{f}_i^{\mathrm{T}}(X_i)d\mathbf{\Lambda}_{ij}\boldsymbol{f}_j(X_j)\right] \tag{11a}$$

$$= \mathbb{E}\left\{\mathrm{tr}\left[\boldsymbol{f}_j(X_j)\boldsymbol{f}_i^{\mathrm{T}}(X_i)d\mathbf{\Lambda}_{ij}\right]\right\}. \tag{11b}$$

Leveraging the Eq. (10), we can derive the partial derivative of term (9a) from Eq. (11b) as:

$$\frac{\partial\,\mathbb{E}\left[\boldsymbol{f}_i^{\mathrm{T}}(X_i)\mathbf{\Lambda}_{ij}\boldsymbol{f}_j(X_j)\right]}{\partial\mathbf{\Lambda}_{ij}} = \mathbb{E}\left[\boldsymbol{f}_j(X_j)\boldsymbol{f}_i^{\mathrm{T}}(X_i)\right]. \tag{12}$$

Similarly, we repeat the same procedure to compute the total differential of second term (9b), which is given by:

$$-\frac{1}{2}d\,\mathrm{tr}\left\{\mathbb{E}\left[\boldsymbol{f}_i(X_i)\boldsymbol{f}_i^{\mathrm{T}}(X_i)\right]\mathbf{\Lambda}_{ij}\mathbb{E}\left[\boldsymbol{f}_j(X_j)\boldsymbol{f}_j^{\mathrm{T}}(X_j)\right]\mathbf{\Lambda}_{ij}\right\}$$

$$= -\frac{1}{2}d\,\mathrm{tr}\left[\mathbf{\Sigma}_{\boldsymbol{f}_i(X_i)}\mathbf{\Lambda}_{ij}\mathbf{\Sigma}_{\boldsymbol{f}_j(X_j)}\mathbf{\Lambda}_{ij}\right] \tag{13a}$$

$$= -\frac{1}{2}\mathrm{tr}\left[\mathbf{\Sigma}_{\boldsymbol{f}_j(X_j)}\mathbf{\Lambda}_{ij}\mathbf{\Sigma}_{\boldsymbol{f}_i(X_i)}d\mathbf{\Lambda}_{ij} + \mathbf{\Sigma}_{\boldsymbol{f}_i(X_i)}\mathbf{\Lambda}_{ij}\mathbf{\Sigma}_{\boldsymbol{f}_j(X_j)}d\mathbf{\Lambda}_{ij}\right], \tag{13b}$$

and then calculate the partial derivative regarding $\mathbf{\Lambda}_{ij}$ using Eq. (10) and (13b) as:

$$-\frac{1}{2}\frac{\partial \operatorname{tr}\left[\mathbf{\Sigma}_{\boldsymbol{f}_i(X_i)}\mathbf{\Lambda}_{ij}\mathbf{\Sigma}_{\boldsymbol{f}_j(X_j)}\mathbf{\Lambda}_{ij}\right]}{\partial \mathbf{\Lambda}_{ij}}$$

$$= -\frac{1}{2}\left\{\left[\mathbf{\Sigma}_{\boldsymbol{f}_j(X_j)}\mathbf{\Lambda}_{ij}\mathbf{\Sigma}_{\boldsymbol{f}_i(X_i)}\right]^{\mathrm{T}} + \left[\mathbf{\Sigma}_{\boldsymbol{f}_i(X_i)}\mathbf{\Lambda}_{ij}\mathbf{\Sigma}_{\boldsymbol{f}_j(X_j)}\right]^{\mathrm{T}}\right\}. \qquad (14)$$

Therefore, by adding up Equation (12) and (14), the derivative of function $\tilde{L}$ is the same as Eq. (1) in Lemma 1.

## C   Algorithms

### C.1   Masked Maximal Correlation Loss

As the masked maximal correlation loss is the negative of $\tilde{L}$ in Eq. (4b), we have:

$$\mathcal{L}_{corr} = -\mathbb{E}\left[\sum_{i\neq j}^{k}\boldsymbol{f}_i^{\mathrm{T}}(X_i)\mathbf{\Lambda}_{ij}\boldsymbol{f}_j(X_j)\right] + \frac{1}{2}\sum_{i\neq j}^{k}\operatorname{tr}\left[\mathbf{\Sigma}_{\boldsymbol{f}_i(X_i)}\mathbf{\Lambda}_{ij}\mathbf{\Sigma}_{\boldsymbol{f}_j(X_j)}\mathbf{\Lambda}_{ij}\right]. \quad (15)$$

Based on Eq. (15), we provide the detailed procedure of masked maximal correlation loss calculation in Algorithm 2.

---

**Algorithm 2.** Calculating the masked maximal correlation loss in one batch

---

**Input**: The feature representations $\boldsymbol{f}$ and $\boldsymbol{g}$ of two modalities $X$ and $Y$ respectively in a batch of size $n$:$\boldsymbol{f}_1(X), \cdots, \boldsymbol{f}_n(X)$ and $\boldsymbol{g}_1(Y), \cdots, \boldsymbol{g}_n(Y)$
**Parameter**: The PCI-mask: $\mathbf{\Lambda}$
**Output**: The correlation loss: $\mathcal{L}_{corr}$

1: Initialize $\mathbf{\Lambda}$
2: Compute the zero-mean features representations:
   $\tilde{\boldsymbol{f}}_i(X) = \boldsymbol{f}_i(X) - \frac{1}{n}\sum_{j=1}^{n}\boldsymbol{f}_j(X), i = 1, \cdots, n$
   $\tilde{\boldsymbol{g}}_i(Y) = \boldsymbol{g}_i(Y) - \frac{1}{n}\sum_{j=1}^{n}\boldsymbol{g}_j(Y), i = 1, \cdots, n$
3: Compute the covariance:
   $\mathbf{\Sigma}_{\tilde{f}} = \frac{1}{n-1}\sum_{i=1}^{n}\tilde{\boldsymbol{f}}_i(X)\tilde{\boldsymbol{f}}_i(X)^{\mathrm{T}}$
   $\mathbf{\Sigma}_{\tilde{g}} = \frac{1}{n-1}\sum_{i=1}^{n}\tilde{\boldsymbol{g}}_i(Y)\tilde{\boldsymbol{g}}_i(Y)^{\mathrm{T}}$
4: Compute the output correlation loss:
   $\mathcal{L}_{corr} = -\frac{1}{n-1}\sum_{i=1}^{n}\tilde{\boldsymbol{f}}_i(X)^{\mathrm{T}}\mathbf{\Lambda}\tilde{\boldsymbol{g}}_i(Y) + \frac{1}{2}tr(\mathbf{\Sigma}_{\tilde{f}}\mathbf{\Lambda}\mathbf{\Sigma}_{\tilde{g}}\mathbf{\Lambda})$

---

### C.2   Routine: Truncation Function

We leverage the truncation function to meet the range constraint in Theorem 1 by projecting the element values in PCI-mask to $[0, 1]$. The routine of the truncation is given by Algorithm 3.

**Algorithm 3.** Projecting values in PCI-mask leveraging truncation

**Input**: PCI-mask: $\Lambda$
**Parameter**: Rank of PCI-mask: $m$
**Output**: Projected PCI-mask: $\bar{\Lambda}$

1: Let $\lambda_i$ in $\Lambda$
2: **for** $i = 1 : m$ **do**
3:    **if** $\lambda_i < 0$ **then**
4:       set $\lambda_i \leftarrow 0$
5:    **else if** $\lambda_i > 1$ **then**
6:       set $\lambda_i \leftarrow 1$
7:    **else**
8:       set $\lambda_i \leftarrow \lambda_i$
9:    **end if**
10: **end for**
11: **return** $\bar{\Lambda} \leftarrow \Lambda$

# D  Supplementary Experiments

## D.1  Implementation Details and Hyperparameters

This section introduces the implementation details and hyper-parameters we used in the experiment. All the experiments are implemented in PyTorch and trained on NVIDIA 2080Ti with fixed hyper-parameter settings. Five-fold cross-validation is adopted while training models on the training dataset. We set the learning rate of the model to 0.0001 and the batch size to 32. The PCI-masks are randomly initialized. When optimizing the PCI-mask, step size $\alpha$ is set to 2, and tolerable error $e$ is set to 0.01 of the sum threshold. We enable the Adam optimizer to train the model and set the maximum number of training epochs as 200. We fixed other grid-searched/Bayesian-optimized [25] hyperparameters during the learning.

## D.2  Experimental Results on BraTS-2015 Dataset

We provide supplementary results on an older version dataset, BraTS-2015, to validate the effectiveness of our proposed approach.

**BraTS-2015 Dataset:** The BraTS-2015 training dataset comprises 220 scans of HGG and 54 scans of LGG, of which four modalities (FLAIR, T1, T1c, and T2) are consistent with BraTS-2020. BraTS-2015 MRI images include four labels: NCR with label 1, ED with label 2, NET with label 3 (which is merged with label 1 in BraTS-2020), and ET with label 4. We perform the same data preprocessing procedure for BraTS-2015.

**Evaluation Metrics:** Besides DSC, Sensitivity, Specificity, and PPV, we add Intersection over Union (IoU), also known as the Jaccard similarity coefficient, as an additional metric for evaluation. IoU measures the overlap of the ground truth and prediction region and is positively correlated to DSC. The

**Table 4.** Segmentation result comparisons between our method and baselines of the best single model on BraTS-2015.

| Baselines | Vanilla U-Net | LSTM U-Net | CI-Autoencoder | U-Net Transformer | Ours |
|---|---|---|---|---|---|
| IoU (NCR) | 0.198 | 0.182 | 0.186 | 0.203 | **0.227** |
| IoU (ED) | 0.386 | 0.395 | 0.435 | 0.537 | **0.612** |
| IoU (NET) | 0.154 | 0.178 | 0.150 | 0.192 | **0.228** |
| IoU (ET) | 0.402 | 0.351 | 0.454 | 0.531 | **0.678** |
| DSC | 0.745 | 0.780 | 0.811 | 0.829 | **0.868** |
| Sensitivity | 0.715 | 0.798 | 0.846 | 0.887 | **0.918** |
| Specificity | 0.998 | 0.999 | 1.000 | 0.999 | **1.000** |
| PPV | 0.712 | 0.738 | 0.864 | 0.853 | **0.891** |

value of IoU ranges from 0 to 1, with 1 signifying the most significant similarity between prediction and ground truth.

**Segmentation Results:** We present the segmentation results of our method on the BraTS-2015 dataset in Table 4, where our method achieves the best results. Specifically, we show the IoU of each label independently, along with DSC, Sensitivity, Specificity, and PPV for the complete tumor labeled by NCR, ED, NET, and ET together. The baselines include the vanilla U-Net [34], LSTM U-Net [40], CI-Autoencoder [23], and U-Net Transformer [32]. In the table, the DSC score of our method outperforms the second-best one by 3.9%, demonstrating the superior performance of our design.

# References

1. Bauer, S., Wiest, R., Nolte, L.P., Reyes, M.: A survey of MRI-based medical image analysis for brain tumor studies. Phys. Med. Biol. **58**(13), R97 (2013)
2. Bian, W., Chen, Y., Ye, X., Zhang, Q.: An optimization-based meta-learning model for MRI reconstruction with diverse dataset. J. Imaging **7**(11), 231 (2021)
3. Bian, W., Zhang, Q., Ye, X., Chen, Y.: A learnable variational model for joint multimodal MRI reconstruction and synthesis. In: Wang, L., Dou, Q., Fletcher, P.T., Speidel, S., Li, S. (eds.) International Conference on Medical Image Computing and Computer-Assisted Intervention, vol. 13436, pp. 354–364. Springer, Cham (2022). https://doi.org/10.1007/978-3-031-16446-0_34
4. Chen, H., Qi, X., Yu, L., Heng, P.A.: DCAN: deep contour-aware networks for accurate gland segmentation. In: Proceedings of the IEEE Conference on Computer Vision and Pattern Recognition, pp. 2487–2496 (2016)
5. Çiçek, Ö., Abdulkadir, A., Lienkamp, S.S., Brox, T., Ronneberger, O.: 3D U-Net: learning dense volumetric segmentation from sparse annotation. In: Ourselin, S., Joskowicz, L., Sabuncu, M.R., Unal, G., Wells, W. (eds.) MICCAI 2016. LNCS, vol. 9901, pp. 424–432. Springer, Cham (2016). https://doi.org/10.1007/978-3-319-46723-8_49
6. Cui, S., Mao, L., Jiang, J., Liu, C., Xiong, S.: Automatic semantic segmentation of brain gliomas from MRI images using a deep cascaded neural network. J. Healthcare Eng. **2018** (2018)

7. DeAngelis, L.M.: Brain tumors. N. Engl. J. Med. **344**(2), 114–123 (2001)
8. Feizi, S., Makhdoumi, A., Duffy, K., Kellis, M., Medard, M.: Network maximal correlation. IEEE Trans. Netw. Sci. Eng. **4**(4), 229–247 (2017)
9. He, K., Zhang, X., Ren, S., Sun, J.: Deep residual learning for image recognition. In: Proceedings of the IEEE Conference on Computer Vision and Pattern Recognition, pp. 770–778 (2016)
10. Huang, G., Liu, Z., Van Der Maaten, L., Weinberger, K.Q.: Densely connected convolutional networks. In: Proceedings of the IEEE Conference on Computer Vision and Pattern Recognition, pp. 4700–4708 (2017)
11. Huang, S.L., Makur, A., Zheng, L., Wornell, G.W.: An information-theoretic approach to universal feature selection in high-dimensional inference. In: 2017 IEEE International Symposium on Information Theory (ISIT), pp. 1336–1340. IEEE (2017)
12. Huang, S.L., Xu, X., Zheng, L.: An information-theoretic approach to unsupervised feature selection for high-dimensional data. IEEE J. Sel. Areas Inf. Theory **1**(1), 157–166 (2020)
13. Huang, S.L., Xu, X., Zheng, L., Wornell, G.W.: An information theoretic interpretation to deep neural networks. In: 2019 IEEE International Symposium on Information Theory (ISIT), pp. 1984–1988. IEEE (2019)
14. Isensee, F., Kickingereder, P., Wick, W., Bendszus, M., Maier-Hein, K.H.: Brain tumor segmentation and radiomics survival prediction: contribution to the BRATS 2017 challenge. In: Crimi, A., Bakas, S., Kuijf, H., Menze, B., Reyes, M. (eds.) BrainLes 2017. LNCS, vol. 10670, pp. 287–297. Springer, Cham (2018). https://doi.org/10.1007/978-3-319-75238-9_25
15. Isensee, F., et al.: Abstract: nnU-Net: self-adapting framework for U-Net-based medical image segmentation. In: Bildverarbeitung für die Medizin 2019. I, pp. 22–22. Springer, Wiesbaden (2019). https://doi.org/10.1007/978-3-658-25326-4_7
16. Jia, H., Cai, W., Huang, H., Xia, Y.: H$^2$NF-net for brain tumor segmentation using multimodal MR imaging: 2nd place solution to BraTS challenge 2020 segmentation task. In: Crimi, A., Bakas, S. (eds.) BrainLes 2020. LNCS, vol. 12659, pp. 58–68. Springer, Cham (2021). https://doi.org/10.1007/978-3-030-72087-2_6
17. Jiang, Z., Ding, C., Liu, M., Tao, D.: Two-stage cascaded U-Net: 1st place solution to BraTS challenge 2019 segmentation task. In: Crimi, A., Bakas, S. (eds.) BrainLes 2019. LNCS, vol. 11992, pp. 231–241. Springer, Cham (2020). https://doi.org/10.1007/978-3-030-46640-4_22
18. Kaganami, H.G., Beiji, Z.: Region-based segmentation versus edge detection. In: 2009 Fifth International Conference on Intelligent Information Hiding and Multimedia Signal Processing, pp. 1217–1221. IEEE (2009)
19. Kingma, D.P., Ba, J.: Adam: a method for stochastic optimization. arXiv preprint arXiv:1412.6980 (2014)
20. Krizhevsky, A., Hinton, G., et al.: Learning multiple layers of features from tiny images (2009)
21. Long, J., Shelhamer, E., Darrell, T.: Fully convolutional networks for semantic segmentation. In: Proceedings of the IEEE Conference on Computer Vision and Pattern Recognition, pp. 3431–3440 (2015)
22. Louis, D.N., et al.: The 2016 world health organization classification of tumors of the central nervous system: a summary. Acta Neuropathol. **131**(6), 803–820 (2016)
23. Ma, F., Zhang, W., Li, Y., Huang, S.L., Zhang, L.: An end-to-end learning approach for multimodal emotion recognition: extracting common and private information. In: 2019 IEEE International Conference on Multimedia and Expo (ICME), pp. 1144–1149. IEEE (2019)

24. McKinley, R., Meier, R., Wiest, R.: Ensembles of densely-connected CNNs with label-uncertainty for brain tumor segmentation. In: Crimi, A., Bakas, S., Kuijf, H., Keyvan, F., Reyes, M., van Walsum, T. (eds.) BrainLes 2018. LNCS, vol. 11384, pp. 456–465. Springer, Cham (2019). https://doi.org/10.1007/978-3-030-11726-9_40

25. Mei, Y., Lan, T., Imani, M., Subramaniam, S.: A Bayesian optimization framework for finding local optima in expensive multi-modal functions. arXiv preprint arXiv:2210.06635 (2022)

26. Menze, B.H., et al.: The multimodal brain tumor image segmentation benchmark (brats). IEEE Trans. Med. Imaging **34**(10), 1993–2024 (2014)

27. Milletari, F., Navab, N., Ahmadi, S.A.: V-Net: fully convolutional neural networks for volumetric medical image segmentation. In: 2016 Fourth International Conference on 3D Vision (3DV), pp. 565–571. IEEE (2016)

28. Muthukrishnan, R., Radha, M.: Edge detection techniques for image segmentation. Int. J. Comput. Sci. Inf. Technol. **3**(6), 259 (2011)

29. Myronenko, A.: 3D MRI brain tumor segmentation using autoencoder regularization. In: Crimi, A., Bakas, S., Kuijf, H., Keyvan, F., Reyes, M., van Walsum, T. (eds.) BrainLes 2018. LNCS, vol. 11384, pp. 311–320. Springer, Cham (2019). https://doi.org/10.1007/978-3-030-11726-9_28

30. Oktay, O., et al.: Attention U-Net: learning where to look for the pancreas. arXiv preprint arXiv:1804.03999 (2018)

31. Pearson, K.: Vii. note on regression and inheritance in the case of two parents. Proc. Roy. Soc. London **58**(347–352), 240–242 (1895)

32. Petit, O., Thome, N., Rambour, C., Themyr, L., Collins, T., Soler, L.: U-Net transformer: self and cross attention for medical image segmentation. In: Lian, C., Cao, X., Rekik, I., Xu, X., Yan, P. (eds.) MLMI 2021. LNCS, vol. 12966, pp. 267–276. Springer, Cham (2021). https://doi.org/10.1007/978-3-030-87589-3_28

33. Rényi, A.: On measures of dependence. Acta Mathematica Academiae Scientiarum Hungarica **10**(3–4), 441–451 (1959)

34. Ronneberger, O., Fischer, P., Brox, T.: U-Net: convolutional networks for biomedical image segmentation. In: Navab, N., Hornegger, J., Wells, W.M., Frangi, A.F. (eds.) MICCAI 2015. LNCS, vol. 9351, pp. 234–241. Springer, Cham (2015). https://doi.org/10.1007/978-3-319-24574-4_28

35. Vaswani, A., et al.: Attention is all you need. In: Advances in Neural Information Processing Systems, pp. 5998–6008 (2017)

36. Wang, G., Li, W., Ourselin, S., Vercauteren, T.: Automatic brain tumor segmentation using cascaded anisotropic convolutional neural networks. In: Crimi, A., Bakas, S., Kuijf, H., Menze, B., Reyes, M. (eds.) BrainLes 2017. LNCS, vol. 10670, pp. 178–190. Springer, Cham (2018). https://doi.org/10.1007/978-3-319-75238-9_16

37. Wang, L., et al.: An efficient approach to informative feature extraction from multimodal data. In: Proceedings of the AAAI Conference on Artificial Intelligence, pp. 5281–5288 (2019)

38. Wang, Y., et al.: Modality-pairing learning for brain tumor segmentation. In: Crimi, A., Bakas, S. (eds.) BrainLes 2020. LNCS, vol. 12658, pp. 230–240. Springer, Cham (2021). https://doi.org/10.1007/978-3-030-72084-1_21

39. Wu, X., Hu, Z., Pei, J., Huang, H.: Serverless federated AUPRC optimization for multi-party collaborative imbalanced data mining. In: SIGKDD Conference on Knowledge Discovery and Data Mining (KDD). ACM (2023)

40. Xu, F., Ma, H., Sun, J., Wu, R., Liu, X., Kong, Y.: LSTM multi-modal UNet for brain tumor segmentation. In: 2019 IEEE 4th International Conference on Image, Vision and Computing (ICIVC), pp. 236–240. IEEE (2019)

41. Xu, X., Huang, S.L.: Maximal correlation regression. IEEE Access **8**, 26591–26601 (2020)

42. Zhang, D., Zhou, F., Jiang, Y., Fu, Z.: MM-BSN: self-supervised image denoising for real-world with multi-mask based on blind-spot network. In: Proceedings of the IEEE/CVF Conference on Computer Vision and Pattern Recognition, pp. 4188–4197 (2023)

43. Zhang, J., Jiang, Z., Dong, J., Hou, Y., Liu, B.: Attention gate ResU-Net for automatic MRI brain tumor segmentation. IEEE Access **8**, 58533–58545 (2020)

44. Zhang, W., Gu, W., Ma, F., Ni, S., Zhang, L., Huang, S.L.: Multimodal emotion recognition by extracting common and modality-specific information. In: Proceedings of the 16th ACM Conference on Embedded Networked Sensor Systems, pp. 396–397 (2018)

45. Zhou, Z., Rahman Siddiquee, M.M., Tajbakhsh, N., Liang, J.: UNet++: a nested U-Net architecture for medical image segmentation. In: Stoyanov, D., et al. (eds.) DLMIA/ML-CDS -2018. LNCS, vol. 11045, pp. 3–11. Springer, Cham (2018). https://doi.org/10.1007/978-3-030-00889-5_1

# Multimodal LLMs for Health Grounded in Individual-Specific Data

Anastasiya Belyaeva[1], Justin Cosentino[1], Farhad Hormozdiari[2], Krish Eswaran[1], Shravya Shetty[1], Greg Corrado[1], Andrew Carroll[1], Cory Y. McLean[2], and Nicholas A. Furlotte[1(✉)]

[1] Google Research, San Francisco, CA 94105, USA
nickfurlotte@google.com
[2] Google Research, Cambridge, MA 02142, USA

**Abstract.** Foundation large language models (LLMs) have shown an impressive ability to solve tasks across a wide range of fields including health. To effectively solve personalized health tasks, LLMs need the ability to ingest a diversity of data modalities that are relevant to an individual's health status. In this paper, we take a step towards creating multimodal LLMs for health that are grounded in individual-specific data by developing a framework (HeLM: Health Large Language Model for Multimodal Understanding) that enables LLMs to use high-dimensional clinical modalities to estimate underlying disease risk. HeLM encodes complex data modalities by learning an encoder that maps them into the LLM's token embedding space and for simple modalities like tabular data by serializing the data into text. Using data from the UK Biobank, we show that HeLM can effectively use demographic and clinical features in addition to high-dimensional time-series data to estimate disease risk. For example, HeLM achieves an AUROC of 0.75 for asthma prediction when combining tabular and spirogram data modalities compared with 0.49 when only using tabular data. Overall, we find that HeLM outperforms or performs at parity with classical machine learning approaches across a selection of eight binary traits. Furthermore, we investigate the downstream uses of this model such as its generalizability to out-of-distribution traits and its ability to power conversations around individual health and wellness.

**Keywords:** Multimodal Large Language Models · Health · UK Biobank

---

A. Belyaeva and J. Cosentino—Equal contribution.
C.Y. McLean and N.A. Furlotte—Equal supervision.

---

**Supplementary Information** The online version contains supplementary material available at https://doi.org/10.1007/978-3-031-47679-2_7.

A. K. Maier et al. (Eds.): ML4MHD 2023, LNCS 14315, pp. 86–102, 2024.
https://doi.org/10.1007/978-3-031-47679-2_7

# 1    Introduction

Foundation large language models (LLMs) have been shown to solve a range of natural language processing (NLP) tasks without having been explicitly trained to do so [4,36]. As a result, researchers are adapting LLMs to solve a variety of non-traditional NLP problems across domains. A recent perspective [23] outlined a variety of health-related use cases that could benefit from foundation LLMs that have not only generalist medical knowledge but that are also infused with individual-specific information such as lab values (e.g., cholesterol and triglycerides), imaging, time-series data, health tracker metrics (e.g., daily step count and heart rate), genome sequences, genetic risk scores, and other omics data modalities. These use cases range from AI clinician assistants to AI-powered early warning systems to user-facing health and wellness chatbots.

While the potential applications for foundation LLMs in health are wide-ranging, at the core of each there is a fundamental need for the model to ingest complex multimodal individual-specific data and use it to gain an understanding of the individual's underlying health risks. The model can then condition responses to queries on the derived risk profile of an individual. Though there has been promising recent work in developing generalist medical LLMs [30–32,38], the problem of using multimodal individual-specific information as context for health-related tasks remains understudied. More broadly, this capability represents one aspect of the general movement towards personalization of LLMs [18,28], which encompasses not only the technical challenges of data integration, but also the complex ethical questions around how the model can and should be used.

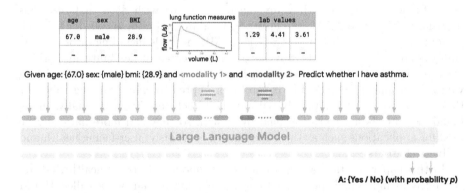

**Fig. 1. Overview of HeLM, a multimodal LLM for health.** Text features (orange) are tokenized and embedded into the token embedding space via a standard embedding matrix. Non-text modalities such as clinical data (blue) or high-dimensional lung function measures (green) are encoded into the same token embedding space via modality-specific encoders. The LLM is tuned to quantify disease risk given complex multimodal inputs. (Color figure online)

Providing relevant health information to an LLM could be as simple as including important disease risk factors, such as lab values, in the prompt by representing these factors as text [10, 16]. Furthermore, in-context learning techniques such as few-shot prompting [4] can be employed by giving the model examples that help it to connect risk factors to underlying disease. However, this solution isn't likely to work for the many complex data modalities found in the health space [1]. For example, it isn't clear how to incorporate images, time-series data, or even rich structured tabular data into the LLM prompt. Furthermore, health factors may not be clearly captured by a single modality but rather may be best predicted by simultaneously incorporating features drawn from multiple modalities.

Recently, a variety of methods have been introduced to extend LLMs to the multimodal setting. The majority of these methods have focused on images and text [2, 17, 21, 24, 25, 39] with some models adding the ability to incorporate diverse modalities, such as the movements of robots, video, and audio [11, 12, 22]. However, these nascent methods have not yet been applied to the health domain. On the other hand, there are a variety of classical machine learning methods for integrating multiple data modalities that are routinely applied in the health domain [1]. Examples include logistic regression classifiers that take multiple modalities as input, various fusion models [19], autoencoder-based models [37], and cross-supervision models [40]. However, these traditional approaches lack several potential advantages when compared to LLM-based methods.

First, foundation LLMs may have encoded extensive prior knowledge about health related traits. For example, an LLM likely understands that hypertension is the same as high blood pressure and may even know something about what number ranges correspond to—normal or high. This prior knowledge can be useful when dealing with heterogeneous data or with data that only has fuzzy labels. Secondly, LLMs can incorporate additional prior knowledge through prompt engineering, whereas in traditional ML methods including priors can be cumbersome. Thirdly, LLMs may have a high degree of flexibility in working with missing data. Whereas traditional methods require imputation of missing values or dropping samples, LLMs can be prompted to ignore missing values or they can be omitted completely without architectural changes. Finally, many foundation LLMs are conversational by design, so they can more naturally be used for applications such as those mentioned previously: user-facing health and wellness chatbots.

In this paper, we take a step towards multimodal LLMs for health that are grounded in individual-specific data by developing a framework called HeLM that enables LLMs to use health-related features to estimate underlying disease risk. The idea is that an LLM with a representation of background risk, can use this as context in answering health-related queries. We formulate a disease classification task and then use the LLM, Flan-PaLMChilla 62b [7], to score potential outcomes. We compare the LLM score with classic supervised machine learning methods such as logistic regression and gradient-boosted decision trees by evaluating their ability to distinguish between individuals with and without the disease.

Using data from the UK Biobank [5], we evaluate different ways of prompting and encoding data and passing it to the LLM to classify disease status. First, we serialize health-related features into text similar to previously proposed approaches [10, 16]. We evaluate zero-shot, few-shot, and a parameter-efficient soft-prompt tuning approach [20]. Generally, we find that the LLM performs better than random in the zero-shot and few-shot cases, and has comparable and often equivalent performance to standard approaches such as logistic regression and a gradient-boosted decision trees (implemented in XGBoost [6]) after prompt tuning. Additionally, for some diseases (e.g., diabetes), the zero-shot and few-shot approaches perform surprisingly well when compared with logistic regression and XGBoost, giving evidence to the model's use of prior knowledge related to disease risk. However, we observe that performance degrades with an increase in the number of input features indicating that the model does not always fully capture signal from serialized text.

To better capture signal from quantitative data, we propose HeLM, a multimodal approach to disease risk estimation based on the PaLM-E framework [11]. In HeLM, non-text modalities are mapped via encoders (trained over input examples) into the same token embedding space as text, where a separate encoder is learned for each modality (see Fig. 1). We show that HeLM matches the performance of classical machine learning methods (logistic regression and XGBoost) and, in some cases, outperforms both the logistic regression and XGBoost models. We show results for encoding tabular data and spirogram curves, a time series representation of lung function used for respiratory disease diagnosis [8, 33]. Finally, we explore how HeLM that has been tuned to quantify disease risk can be used in downstream conversational tasks. Here, we find that conversational ability degrades in the tuned LLM, which is consistent with what others have reported [35]. We discuss future directions such as fine-tuning schemes that may mitigate degradation.

## 2    Methods

### 2.1    LLMs with Tabular Data

An individual's health status is often represented by a set of values stored in tabular format. We explore whether serializing tabular data into natural language and passing the resulting text to the LLM (Flan-PaLMChilla 62b [7]) is sufficient to achieve strong predictive performance. We construct serialized inputs by mapping table column names and corresponding values into JSON-like format, which is combined with the base prompt. For example, for diabetes prediction, we formulate the following sentence using the data: *"Predict if a patient has the condition or not. bmi: {28.9}. age: {67.0}. sex: {male}. diabetes: {"*. We then compute the log-likelihood of the sentence being completed with *"yes}"* or *"no}"*. This log-likelihood serves as a risk score and can be evaluated using metrics such as AUROC and AUPRC to assess discriminatory power.

We evaluate the LLM's performance in the zero-shot, few-shot and soft-prompt tuning settings. In the zero-shot setting, the serialized text input is given directly to the model. In this case, the LLM heavily leverages prior knowledge. In the few-shot scenario, we prefix 10 examples randomly sampled from the training dataset to the model's prompt. For soft-prompt tuning, following [20], we learn a soft prompt to condition the frozen language model to perform well on the diseases of interest.

Briefly, soft-prompt tuning is a parameter efficient tuning technique that's commonly used to steer the frozen LLM to perform well on a downstream task given labeled data. Instead of fine-tuning the weights of the LLM or forming a hard prompt out of tokens as in the few-shot scenario, soft-prompt tuning learns a matrix $P \subset \mathbb{R}^{p \times k}$ in the token embedding space, where $p$ is the length of the prompt and $k$ is the size of the language embedding space. The soft-prompt $P$ is then concatenated with the embedded tokens and passed to the decoder. We train the soft-prompt using pairs of examples $(X, Y)$ and backpropagation to update the soft-prompt with the goal of maximizing the probability of $Y$. We train for 20,000 steps and use 1000 training examples.

## 2.2 Multimodal LLMs for Health: HeLM

To enable the LLM to reason over complex high-dimensional inputs, we embed non-text data modalities, including time-series data like spirograms and tabular data, into the same latent space as the language tokens (see Fig. 1). We use separate encoders for each non-text data modality, where each encoder learns a mapping to the token embedding space. This approach is based on the PaLM-E framework [11]. All of the inputs are then processed together by a pre-trained LLM. More precisely, LLMs typically tokenize the words in a sentence and map the resulting tokens $w_i$ into a language embedding space $\mathcal{X} \subset \mathbb{R}^k$ via a large embedding matrix $x_i = \gamma(w_i)$ where $\gamma : \mathcal{W} \to \mathcal{X}$. In HeLM, non-text modalities are mapped to a sequence of vectors in $\mathcal{X}$ via encoders. For example, for mapping the spirogram time-series we trained $\phi_s : \mathcal{S} \to \mathcal{X}^{q_s}$ encoder and for mapping tabular data we trained $\phi_t : \mathcal{T} \to \mathcal{X}^{q_t}$ encoder, where $q_s$ and $q_t$ correspond to the number of vectors in $\mathcal{X}$ space or in other words how many "multimodal" tokens each modality is mapped to. We set $q_s = 6$ and $q_t = 6$ for all experiments, however in general these can be treated as tunable hyper-parameters. In summary, each vector $x_i$ is formed from either the token embedder $\gamma$ or a modality-specific encoder:

$$
x_i = \begin{cases} \gamma(w_i) & \text{if } i \text{ is a text token} \\ \phi_s(s_i) & \text{if } i \text{ corresponds to the spirogram modality} \\ \phi_t(t_i) & \text{if } i \text{ corresponds to the tabular modality} \end{cases}
$$

Non-text and text modalities can be injected in any order. We train the modality-specific encoders keeping the pre-trained LLM weights frozen. This is similar to soft-prompt tuning but conditioned on data from a specific modality.

For experiments considering multiple diseases we train a single HeLM model on a mixture of all diseases as opposed to one model per disease.

### 2.3 UK Biobank Dataset Preparation

We obtain clinical features, spirometry, and disease labels from the UK Biobank (UKB) [5]. Similar to previous work, we focus on the European genetic ancestry subpopulation [3]. Limiting to European ancestry within the UK Biobank is a standard heuristic for reducing phenotypic heterogeneity, due to the correlation between population structure and phenotypic variation [9]. Differences in phenotypes across ancestries are multifactorial—socio-economic, cultural, etc.—but are often highly correlated with genetic background and thus population structure. Therefore, selecting study individuals based on a single genetic background is a convenient way to reduce heterogeneity in underlying disease risk, at the expense of creating bias in the dataset and subsequent analyses that utilize this data.

We defined binary phenotype labels using medical records comprising ICD-9 hospital inpatient (HESIN) billing codes, ICD-10 primary care and general practitioner (GP) read codes, and self-report data. Diseases include asthma, diabetes, hypertension, stroke, myocardial infarction, major depression, migraine, all cause mortality, cataracts, gastroesophageal reflux disease (GERD), hay fever eczema (atopic eczema), osteoarthritis, and pneumonia. The following clinical features, lab values, and self-reported statuses sourced from questionnaires were used as model inputs: age, sex, body mass index (BMI), high-density lipoprotein (HDL) cholesterol, low-density lipoprotein (LDL) cholesterol, total cholesterol, triglycerides, diastolic blood pressure, smoking status, snoring, insomnia, daytime napping, average nightly sleeping, and chronotype. See table S1 for details describing feature definitions.

Spirometry data was prepared following the preprocessing procedures outlined in [8]. In short, we used raw volumetric flow curves containing exhalation volume sampled at 10 ms intervals to liters and then computed the corresponding flow curve by approximating the first derivative with respect to time by taking a finite difference. The volume-time and flow-time curves were then normalized to length 1,000 and combined to generate a one-dimensional flow-volume spirogram. Following well-accepted spirometry quality control standards, we filter the dataset to individuals with at least one acceptable blow from the first visit [8,27,29].

We randomly partitioned patients with valid data entries for all phenotype labels and clinical features into distinct training and validation datasets.

## 3    Experimental Results

We present LLM risk prediction performance across eight disease classification tasks under varied experimental settings. We begin by assessing the effectiveness of zero-shot and few-shot prompting as well as soft-prompt tuning on a pre-trained foundation model using health data serialized into text. We then demonstrate that directly mapping quantitative features into the LLM's latent token space significantly improves model performance. Finally, using asthma as a case study, we show that this mapping procedure generalizes to high-dimensional lung function data.

### 3.1   Quantifying Disease Risk Using Zero-Shot, Few-Shot, and Soft-Prompt Tuning

We first establish a baseline for LLM disease risk prediction using zero-shot, few-shot, and soft-prompt tuning with a frozen Flan-PaLMChilla 62b model [7]. We define classification tasks using a diverse set of binary phenotype targets (see Sect. 2.3). For each task and prompting method, we evaluate a "baseline" set of model inputs consisting of age, sex, and BMI as well as an "expanded" set that includes eleven additional clinical and wellness traits: HDL cholesterol, LDL cholesterol, total cholesterol, total triglycerides, diastolic blood pressure, smoking status, average sleep duration, insomnia, snoring, daytime napping, and chronotype (i.e., whether a patient is a morning or evening person). These predictors were chosen based on prior knowledge that they should be informative about the selected targets.

We score a validation dataset ($n = 3,000$) using the methodology outlined in Sect. 2. For each validation sample, we generate a disease risk score by computing the log probability of a positive disease label. Similarly, to obtain the logistic regression and XGBoost scores, we compute the probability of a positive disease label given the respective model fit on a separate training set ($n = 10,000$).

Table 1 shows performance for each prompting method and input set compared to the baseline models. We observe that at least one prompting technique is competitive with the baselines for most tasks. In some cases (e.g., hypertension and diabetes), zero-shot and few-shot models perform surprisingly well despite seeing little to no training data compared to the baselines, an observation also made by [16]. This suggests that the LLM uses prior knowledge about the relationships between age, sex, BMI and disease likelihood.

Focusing on the baseline feature set (age, sex, and BMI), we aimed to understand how the LLM derives scores. We estimated the importance of each input feature by regressing the features against the scores output by the model. Coefficients from the linear regression model are used to measure feature importance and concordance across methods. Figure S1 shows the result of this analysis for four traits. For diabetes, hypertension, and stroke, we see concordance between logistic regression, XGBoost and the LLM models in terms of direction and relative magnitude of effects. Additionally, we find a strong correlation between logistic regression and LLM scores (Spearman = 0.46–0.93 across prompting methods), while the correlation between LLM and XGBoost scores is weaker (Spearman = 0.39–0.65). On the other hand, for migraine, we see little concordance in direction and relative magnitude of effects for zero-shot and few-shot LLMs, indicating that the LLM doesn't have sufficient prior knowledge to relate migraine with the input features. However, this is corrected in the soft-prompt case, where we see concordance and high Spearman correlation between soft-prompt tuned LLM and logistic regression (0.85). On the other hand, the soft-prompt tuned LLM has low Spearman correlation with XGBoost (0.31), which is a non-linear model. Given this, we hypothesize that the LLM is effectively scoring outcomes using what translates to a simple linear function of the input features and that this linear mapping is effectively learned via soft-prompting.

**Table 1. Comparison of AUC and AUPRC between LLM-based classifiers and classical machine learning approaches on the validation set.** The models with "baseline" input features use age, sex and BMI as model features, while the models with the "expanded" set also include 11 additional clinical and wellness traits. The mean AUC/AUPRC and the corresponding 95% confidence intervals were calculated across 1,000 bootstrapping iterations. Bold cells denote the best models for a given phenotype and input feature set, where statistical significance is determined via paired bootstrapping. Logistic regression and XGBoost models were trained on 10,000 samples, few-shot on 10 samples and soft-prompt tuning on 1,000 samples.

| Phenotype | Model | Baseline AUC | Expanded AUC | Baseline AUPRC | Expanded AUPRC |
|---|---|---|---|---|---|
| All Cause Mortality (prevalence = 6.83%) | Zero-shot | 0.61 (0.57–0.64) | 0.61 (0.57–0.65) | 0.10 (0.08–0.12) | 0.11 (0.09–0.14) |
| | Few-shot | 0.65 (0.61–0.69) | 0.65 (0.61–0.69) | 0.12 (0.10–0.15) | **0.12 (0.09–0.15)** |
| | Soft-prompt | **0.69 (0.66–0.73)** | **0.69 (0.65–0.72)** | 0.13 (0.10–0.16) | **0.14 (0.11–0.18)** |
| | LogReg | **0.71 (0.67–0.74)** | 0.68 (0.64–0.72) | **0.15 (0.12–0.19)** | **0.16 (0.13–0.21)** |
| | XGBoost | 0.67 (0.62–0.70) | **0.67 (0.62–0.70)** | 0.13 (0.10–0.17) | 0.13 (0.10–0.17) |
| Diabetes (prevalence = 7.60%) | Zero-shot | 0.70 (0.67–0.73) | 0.61 (0.57–0.65) | 0.18 (0.14–0.23) | 0.12 (0.10–0.15) |
| | Few-shot | 0.72 (0.69–0.76) | 0.67 (0.64–0.70) | **0.19 (0.15–0.24)** | 0.14 (0.11–0.17) |
| | Soft-prompt | 0.72 (0.69–0.76) | 0.68 (0.64–0.72) | **0.23 (0.18–0.28)** | 0.17 (0.14–0.22) |
| | LogReg | **0.74 (0.70–0.77)** | **0.75 (0.72–0.79)** | **0.23 (0.18–0.28)** | **0.26 (0.21–0.32)** |
| | XGBoost | 0.73 (0.69–0.76) | 0.73 (0.69–0.76) | **0.22 (0.18–0.27)** | 0.22 (0.17–0.26) |
| Hypertension (prevalence = 40.03%) | Zero-shot | 0.70 (0.68–0.72) | 0.68 (0.66–0.70) | 0.60 (0.56–0.62) | 0.57 (0.54–0.60) |
| | Few-shot | 0.73 (0.71–0.75) | 0.72 (0.70–0.73) | 0.62 (0.59–0.64) | 0.59 (0.56–0.62) |
| | Soft-prompt | 0.72 (0.70–0.74) | 0.72 (0.70–0.74) | 0.60 (0.57–0.63) | 0.59 (0.56–0.62) |
| | LogReg | 0.74 (0.72–0.76) | 0.74 (0.72–0.76) | 0.63 (0.60–0.66) | **0.65 (0.62–0.68)** |
| | XGBoost | **0.77 (0.75–0.78)** | **0.77 (0.75–0.78)** | **0.66 (0.63–0.69)** | 0.66 (0.63–0.69) |
| Major Depression (prevalence = 13.03%) | Zero-shot | 0.54 (0.51–0.57) | 0.58 (0.55–0.61) | 0.15 (0.13–0.17) | 0.17 (0.14–0.19) |
| | Few-shot | 0.50 (0.47–0.53) | 0.55 (0.52–0.58) | 0.14 (0.12–0.15) | 0.15 (0.13–0.17) |
| | Soft-prompt | **0.60 (0.57–0.63)** | 0.47 (0.44–0.50) | **0.20 (0.17–0.23)** | 0.12 (0.11–0.14) |
| | LogReg | **0.60 (0.57–0.63)** | 0.62 (0.59–0.65) | 0.19 (0.16–0.22) | **0.19 (0.17–0.22)** |
| | XGBoost | 0.54 (0.52–0.57) | 0.54 (0.52–0.57) | 0.16 (0.14–0.18) | 0.16 (0.14–0.18) |
| Migraine (prevalence = 3.77%) | Zero-shot | 0.51 (0.45–0.56) | 0.49 (0.45–0.55) | 0.05 (0.03–0.07) | 0.04 (0.03–0.05) |
| | Few-shot | 0.45 (0.40–0.50) | 0.47 (0.42–0.53) | 0.03 (0.03–0.04) | 0.03 (0.03–0.04) |
| | Soft-prompt | **0.64 (0.59–0.69)** | 0.51 (0.46–0.56) | **0.07 (0.05–0.09)** | 0.04 (0.03–0.06) |
| | LogReg | **0.62 (0.56–0.68)** | 0.62 (0.56–0.67) | 0.07 (0.04–0.11) | 0.06 (0.04–0.08) |
| | XGBoost | 0.60 (0.54–0.66) | 0.60 (0.54–0.66) | 0.06 (0.04–0.07) | 0.06 (0.04–0.07) |
| Myocardial Infarction (prevalence = 5.93%) | Zero-shot | 0.61 (0.57–0.65) | 0.61 (0.56–0.65) | 0.08 (0.06–0.10) | 0.09 (0.07–0.12) |
| | Few-shot | 0.67 (0.63–0.71) | 0.65 (0.61–0.68) | **0.11 (0.09–0.14)** | 0.10 (0.08–0.12) |
| | Soft-prompt | **0.71 (0.67–0.74)** | 0.68 (0.64–0.71) | 0.12 (0.10–0.15) | 0.11 (0.09–0.14) |
| | LogReg | **0.71 (0.67–0.74)** | 0.70 (0.65–0.74) | 0.12 (0.09–0.15) | **0.16 (0.12–0.21)** |
| | XGBoost | 0.69 (0.65–0.73) | 0.69 (0.65–0.73) | 0.14 (0.11–0.19) | 0.14 (0.11–0.19) |
| Stroke (prevalence = 4.00%) | Zero-shot | 0.61 (0.56–0.66) | 0.55 (0.49–0.60) | 0.06 (0.05–0.09) | 0.05 (0.04–0.06) |
| | Few-shot | 0.65 (0.60–0.69) | 0.60 (0.56–0.65) | 0.07 (0.05–0.09) | 0.05 (0.04–0.07) |
| | Soft-prompt | 0.63 (0.58–0.68) | 0.50 (0.45–0.55) | **0.09 (0.06–0.12)** | 0.05 (0.03–0.06) |
| | LogReg | **0.69 (0.64–0.74)** | **0.73 (0.68–0.77)** | 0.10 (0.07–0.14) | **0.14 (0.09–0.19)** |
| | XGBoost | **0.68 (0.63–0.72)** | 0.68 (0.63–0.72) | **0.09 (0.06–0.12)** | 0.09 (0.06–0.12) |

In the expanded feature set, we often find that the LLM with zero-shot prompting has poorer performance (e.g., on diabetes) when compared with the LLM with zero-shot prompting using the smaller feature set. This may indicate that the LLM has insufficient prior knowledge about the features contained in the expanded set. However, unlike the baseline features, the model is not able to match baseline performance even when using soft-prompt tuning. This indicates that for a complex set of input features, text serialization does not yield a representation that fully captures the available signal. Together, these results motivate the use of a multimodal approach to directly embed quantitative data into the prompt.

### 3.2  Encoding Quantitative Data Using HeLM

To assess the benefit of directly embedding quantitative data into the LLM's latent token space, we repeat the experiments from Sect. 3.1 but encode the "extended" inputs using the HeLM framework. We learn an encoder $\phi_t$, an MLP (two hidden layers of size 1024 and 4096, respectively), that takes as input quantitative features and maps them into the embedding space. We train this model over a mixture of all seven binary traits ($n = 10,000$ for each trait).

Table 2 shows performance metrics for HeLM compared with logistic regression and XGBoost. We see that by directly encoding the tabular data into token space, HeLM performs at parity with the best baseline methods and for all cause mortality, hypertension and myocardial infarction HeLM outperforms the best baseline. In comparing the scoring methods, we again find that HeLM scores are highly correlated with logistic regression scores (Spearman = 0.70–0.87; Figure S4a–Figure S5c). In Figure S2, we repeat the feature importance analysis, this time comparing HeLM with logistic regression and XGBoost. Similar to Sect. 3.1, we see strong concordance between feature weights, particularly for features that have the most importance. Taken together, these results are consistent with our previous hypothesis that the LLM scores outcomes in a way that is highly consistent with logistic regression and that the LLM is arriving at these scores by similarly linearly weighting input features.

In the case of hypertenion, we see that HeLM significantly outperforms logistic regression and XGBoost, while XGBoost appears to have a slight advantage over logistic regression. In addition, the HeLM score is more correlated with the XGBoost score when compared with logistic (Spearman 0.87 vs. 0.76), which is not the case for any of the other traits. Although, in no way conclusive, this may indicate that by mapping the tabular data into embedding space, the LLM takes advantage of non-linear relationships between input features and hypertension. This phenomenon may account for some of the cases where HeLM outperforms the baseline methods.

We hypothesized that HeLM has an advantage over logistic regression due to being trained over a mixture of traits and thus benefiting from transfer learning across traits. To evaluate this, we selected three traits (hypertension, all cause mortality and myocardial infarction) where HeLM performed better than logistic regression in terms of AUROC. For each, we trained a single task HeLM (a separate model for each trait) and compared with the mixture. Overall, we see that the mixture trained HeLM does not have an advantage over the single task model (Table S2). Training on a mixture of diseases is still advantageous since it yields a single model that can be used for a variety of diseases as opposed to separate models for each disease (as is the case for logistic regression and XGBoost).

### 3.3   Estimating Asthma Risk Using Multiple Modalities

Using HeLM to leverage tabular data clearly showed that this is a promising direction for quantifying disease risk. Next, we evaluate whether HeLM can incorporate more complex data modalities such as a spirogram, a time-series curve which measures the amount of air an individual can breath in and out

**Table 2. Comparison of AUC and AUPRC between a HeLM, logistic regression and XGBoost models on the validation set.** The binary phenotypes are predicted from the 14 "expanded set" input features from Table 1. The features are both encoded in text as in Table 1 and also included as a secondary quantitative data modality.

| Phenotype | Model | AUC | AUPRC |
|---|---|---|---|
| All Cause Mortality | HeLM | **0.71 (0.68–0.75)** | **0.18 (0.14–0.23)** |
| | LogReg | 0.68 (0.64–0.72) | **0.16 (0.13–0.21)** |
| | XGBoost | 0.67 (0.62–0.70) | 0.13 (0.10–0.17) |
| Diabetes | HeLM | **0.77 (0.74–0.80)** | **0.27 (0.22–0.33)** |
| | LogReg | **0.75 (0.72–0.79)** | **0.26 (0.21–0.32)** |
| | XGBoost | 0.73 (0.69–0.76) | 0.22 (0.17–0.26) |
| Hypertension | HeLM | **0.79 (0.77–0.81)** | **0.69 (0.66–0.72)** |
| | LogReg | 0.74 (0.72–0.76) | 0.65 (0.62–0.68) |
| | XGBoost | 0.77 (0.75–0.78) | 0.66 (0.63–0.69) |
| Major Depression | HeLM | **0.63 (0.60–0.65)** | **0.19 (0.17–0.22)** |
| | LogReg | **0.62 (0.59–0.65)** | **0.19 (0.17–0.22)** |
| | XGBoost | 0.54 (0.52–0.57) | 0.16 (0.14–0.18) |
| Migraine | HeLM | **0.61 (0.55–0.66)** | **0.06 (0.04–0.07)** |
| | LogReg | **0.62 (0.56–0.67)** | **0.06 (0.04–0.08)** |
| | XGBoost | **0.60 (0.54–0.66)** | **0.06 (0.04–0.07)** |
| Myocardial Infarction | HeLM | **0.73 (0.69–0.77)** | **0.15 (0.12–0.19)** |
| | LogReg | 0.70 (0.65–0.74) | **0.16 (0.12–0.21)** |
| | XGBoost | 0.69 (0.65–0.73) | **0.14 (0.11–0.19)** |
| Stroke | HeLM | **0.73 (0.68–0.77)** | **0.14 (0.09–0.20)** |
| | LogReg | **0.73 (0.68–0.77)** | **0.14 (0.09–0.19)** |
| | XGBoost | 0.68 (0.63–0.72) | 0.09 (0.06–0.12) |

of their lungs. Spirometry is commonly used to assess pulmonary function and the presence of respiratory diseases. Thus, we focus on the task of quantifying asthma risk.

To this end, we trained a HeLM model with three modalities as input: tabular data (14 "expanded set" input features) as well as spirometry, along with tabular data serialized to text. We do not include a textual description of the spirogram since it's unclear how to summarize this data in text. We encode spirometry data into the token embedding space via a one-dimensional variant of the ResNet18 architecture [14,15], followed by an MLP (two hidden layers of size 1024 and 4096, respectively). We use a pre-trained model from [8] for the ResNet18 part of the encoder and only update the weights of the MLP. The ResNet18 model was trained to predict asthma and COPD. We take as input the 128-dimensional embedding, corresponding to the penultimate layer. Similar to Sect. 3.2, we use an MLP to encode tabular data into the token embedding space.

The model is instructed to predict asthma using supervised labels ("yes" or "no") as targets in training. We trained on $n = 16,724$ samples from the UK Biobank, which were obtained by subsampling the dataset to achieve a one-to-one case-control class distribution to ensure a balanced representation of categories. As a direct baseline, we also trained a model that linearly combined the 128-dimensional embedding from the ResNet18 model and tabular data, which we term ResNet18 1D (tabular data + spirogram).

In order to assess whether the multimodal HeLM model is leveraging the additional spirogram modality for asthma prediction, we trained several models on tabular data only, without the spirogram. Following Sect. 3.2 we trained a logistic regression model, XGBoost, an LLM with soft-prompt tuning and HeLM using tabular data only.

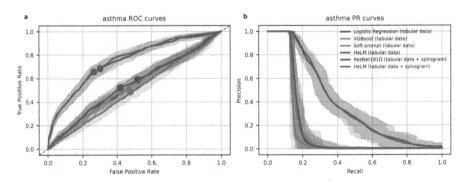

**Fig. 2. Inclusion of additional input modalities improves HeLM asthma detection.** (a) ROC and (b) Precision-recall (PR) for asthma phenotype prediction using tabular data only versus tabular data and spirometry. We compare HeLM, ResNet18 1D, logistic regression, XGBoost, and a soft-prompt tuned LLM trained on either a single modality (tabular) or two modalities (tabular and spirometry).

Figure 2 shows the model performance on a held-out set of individuals with valid spirograms ($n = 2,289$). We observe that the HeLM model trained on two non-text modalities (tabular data and spirogram) is successfully leveraging the additional spirogram modality to boost the performance on asthma prediction. For example, the AUROC (AUPRC) increases from $0.49 \pm 0.02$ ($0.14 \pm 0.01$) for the LLM trained on tabular data only via soft-prompt tuning to $0.75 \pm 0.01$ ($0.38 \pm 0.02$) for HeLM trained on tabular data and a spirogram. The comparison with soft-prompt tuned LLM on tabular data is particularly important since it is the only other method that can also generate natural language text and thus provide recommendations, answer questions, and summarize given an individual's health context. We also observe that HeLM trained on tabular and spirogram data performs on par with the linear combination of the ResNet181D model on spirogram and tabular data.

### 3.4    Using HeLM for Out-of-Distribution Traits

Deep learning methods have shown significant performance degradation when applied to out-of-distribution (OOD) data [26]. We investigated HeLM OOD performance by applying it to a set of traits not in the training set. Considering cataract, gastroesophageal reflux disease (GERD), hay fever eczema (atopic eczema), osteoarthritis, and pneumonia, we compared HeLM with trait-specific logistic regression models (Table 3). We observed that HeLM (not trained on the trait) performs on par with logistic regression (trained on the trait) in four out of five of the tested traits. Taken at face-value this implies that HeLM is leveraging prior information about the impact of risk factors on disease learned from related traits in the training data. However, to truly understand how the model arrives at the OOD scores, will take additional research.

### 3.5    Natural Language Generation

Finally, we assess whether an LLM can incorporate multimodal data to tailor conversational tasks. Approximating a two-stage approach in which a model is trained to quantify risk and then trained to use these risk estimates in conversational tasks, we first use HeLM to compute asthma risk from a spirogram embedding and encode the predicted risk as text into the PaLM-2 model [13] for exercise recommendations: *"I have a p% chance of having asthma. What are some exercises you would suggest, given this information? Please tailor your recommendations to my health status."* Over 110 examples that span the asthma risk spectrum we observe differential recommendations based on predicted asthma risk (Figure S3).

This approach is inefficient as it requires transforming risk predictions back to the textual domain. Ideally, the LLM should condition recommendations directly upon the embedded multimodal data. To this end, we qualitatively explore the natural language generation capability of a HeLM model trained for the asthma task: *"Let's think step by step. Given the following spirogram:⟨spirogram⟩, do they have asthma? Based on that what is the most recommended exercise?"*. A

**Table 3. Comparison of AUC and AUPRC between zero-shot, few-shot LLM-based classifiers, HeLM and a logistic regression model on the validation set in OOD setting.** While logistic regression models were trained on the data for the trait, HeLM was not trained for the trait. The binary phenotypes are predicted from the 14 "expanded set" input features from Table 1. The features are both encoded in text as in Table 1 and also included as a secondary quantitative data modality. "prev" denotes prevalence.

| Phenotype | Model | AUC | AUPRC |
|---|---|---|---|
| Cataract (prev = 13.51%) | Zero-shot | 0.58 (0.55–0.61) | 0.17 (0.15–0.20) |
| | Few-shot | 0.63 (0.60–0.65) | 0.18 (0.16–0.20) |
| | HeLM | **0.71 (0.69–0.73)** | 0.24 (0.21–0.27) |
| | LogReg | **0.72 (0.69–0.74)** | **0.27 (0.23–0.31)** |
| GERD (prev = 17.33%) | Zero-shot | 0.58 (0.55–0.60) | 0.22 (0.19–0.25) |
| | Few-shot | 0.57 (0.54–0.60) | 0.21 (0.18–0.23) |
| | HeLM | **0.61 (0.59–0.64)** | **0.25 (0.22–0.28)** |
| | LogReg | **0.61 (0.59–0.64)** | **0.26 (0.23–0.29)** |
| Hay Fever Eczema (prev = 23.84%) | Zero-shot | 0.48 (0.46–0.51) | 0.23 (0.21–0.24) |
| | Few-shot | 0.46 (0.44–0.49) | 0.23 (0.21–0.25) |
| | HeLM | 0.47 (0.44–0.49) | 0.22 (0.20–0.24) |
| | LogReg | **0.57 (0.55–0.60)** | **0.28 (0.26–0.31)** |
| Osteoarthritis (prev = 28.13%) | Zero-shot | 0.60 (0.58–0.62) | 0.36 (0.33–0.39) |
| | Few-shot | 0.63 (0.61–0.65) | 0.38 (0.35–0.40) |
| | HeLM | **0.65 (0.63–0.67)** | 0.41 (0.38–0.44) |
| | LogReg | **0.67 (0.65–0.69)** | **0.44 (0.40–0.47)** |
| Pneumonia (prev = 6.50%) | Zero-shot | 0.56 (0.52–0.60) | 0.08 (0.06–0.10) |
| | Few-shot | 0.59 (0.55–0.63) | 0.08 (0.07–0.10) |
| | HeLM | **0.68 (0.65–0.72)** | **0.16 (0.12–0.21)** |
| | LogReg | **0.67 (0.63–0.71)** | **0.16 (0.12–0.20)** |

sample answer for an individual with asthma is *"low intensity aerobic exercise. The answer: yes."* and for an individual without asthma *"Swimming. The answer: no."*. We observe that while the model gives sample exercise recommendations that are reasonable (e.g., a low intensity exercise for someone with asthma), it also learned to include yes/no in its answer. This is likely because it has associated our particular question/answer format with the presence of multimodal tokens. The risk prediction results demonstrated that the model can learn to operate on spirograms in the token space, so we expect that including more diverse input and output pairs and generative tasks may improve conversational ability and plan to explore this in future work.

# 4   Discussion

Grounding LLMs in individual-specific information is required to create personalized experiences across a large set of applications. Effective application in health presents unique challenges owing to the high-dimensional and multimodal nature of relevant input data that do not clearly map into text. In this paper, we defined a framework (HeLM) for mapping non-text data modalities into token embedding space and providing this information as context for a foundation LLM to perform disease risk prediction. Using data from the UK Biobank, we showed that HeLM is competitive with classic ML approaches and that—in some cases—the LLM outperforms these methods. The results highlight the promise of enabling LLMs to quantify underlying health risks by leveraging complex multimodal health data.

While these results demonstrate the effectiveness of a multimodal approach, there are many extensions to explore in future work. Though we have focused solely on scalar lab values and high-dimensional lung function data, biobanks contain individual-level data spanning a wide array of clinical modalities. An immediate next step is exploring the effectiveness of simultaneously embedding additional imaging data, such as fundus images or cardiac MRI, in a single input prompt to better understand how jointly modeling such inputs impacts predictive power. Additionally, this experimental setting motivates the study of how an LLM handles missing data and whether the model could "impute" predictive signal from various modality combinations. Furthermore, we have only explored whether an LLM can learn to *understand* non-text data, but have not assessed whether a similar approach can *generate* non-text-based outputs.

A major question that arises from this work is whether enabling LLMs to use multimodal data for health risk prediction can improve their ability to provide relevant personalized suggestions. To this end, we experimented with using HeLM to offer health-related recommendations that are conditioned on an understanding of risk. However, we found that conversational ability degraded after model tuning. This is consistent with previous observations [35], though there is some evidence that larger models are more robust to degradation [11].

In addition, it will be important for conversational agents to explain why they placed individuals into high or low risk categories, and to quantify their level of uncertainty. Alignment issues are also keenly important, as some health-related topics are sensitive and complex to explain, lack expert consensus for best practices, or are sensitive to the culture and preferences of the user.

Finally, LLM-based models that have been trained on available health-related data to quantify disease may show differential performance across demographic groups due to computational, systemic, and human biases [34]. Evaluation and mitigation of this is key to avoid perpetuating and increasing existing health disparities. These are complex issues that we have not attempted to address in this work, but will be extremely important to address before deploying multimodal LLMs for health.

**Acknowledgements.** The authors would like to thank Katrin Tomanek for providing software, inspiration, and know-how that influenced the direction of this work. We also thank Ted Yun for helpful discussions and feedback.

# References

1. Acosta, J.N., Falcone, G.J., Rajpurkar, P., Topol, E.J.: Multimodal biomedical AI. Nat. Med. **28**(9), 1773–1784 (2022)
2. Alayrac, J.B., et al.: Flamingo: a visual language model for few-shot learning. In: Advances in Neural Information Processing Systems, vol. 35, pp. 23716–23736 (2022)
3. Alipanahi, B., et al.: Large-scale machine-learning-based phenotyping significantly improves genomic discovery for optic nerve head morphology. Am. J. Hum. Genet. **108**(7), 1217–1230 (2021)
4. Brown, T., et al.: Language models are few-shot learners. In: Advances in Neural Information Processing Systems, vol. 33, pp. 1877–1901 (2020)
5. Bycroft, C., et al.: The UK Biobank resource with deep phenotyping and genomic data. Nature **562**(7726), 203–209 (2018)
6. Chen, T., Guestrin, C.: XGBoost: a scalable tree boosting system. In: Proceedings of the 22nd ACM SIGKDD International Conference on Knowledge Discovery and Data Mining, KDD 2016, pp. 785–794. ACM, New York (2016). https://doi.org/10.1145/2939672.2939785
7. Chung, H.W., et al.: Scaling instruction-finetuned language models. arXiv preprint arXiv:2210.11416 (2022)
8. Cosentino, J., et al.: Inference of chronic obstructive pulmonary disease with deep learning on raw spirograms identifies new genetic loci and improves risk models. Nat. Genet. **55**, 787–795 (2023)
9. Diaz-Papkovich, A., Anderson-Trocmé, L., Ben-Eghan, C., Gravel, S.: UMAP reveals cryptic population structure and phenotype heterogeneity in large genomic cohorts. PLoS Genet. **15**(11), e1008432 (2019)
10. Dinh, T., et al.: LIFT: language-interfaced fine-tuning for non-language machine learning tasks. In: Advances in Neural Information Processing Systems, vol. 35, pp. 11763–11784 (2022)
11. Driess, D., et al.: PaLM-E: an embodied multimodal language model. arXiv preprint arXiv:2303.03378 (2023)
12. Girdhar, R., et al.: ImageBind: one embedding space to bind them all. arXiv preprint arXiv:2305.05665 (2023)
13. Google: PaLM 2 technical report. arXiv preprint arXiv:2305.10403 (2023)
14. He, K., Zhang, X., Ren, S., Sun, J.: Deep residual learning for image recognition. In: Proceedings of the IEEE Conference on Computer Vision and Pattern Recognition, pp. 770–778 (2016)
15. He, T., Zhang, Z., Zhang, H., Zhang, Z., Xie, J., Li, M.: Bag of tricks for image classification with convolutional neural networks. In: Proceedings of the IEEE/CVF Conference on Computer Vision and Pattern Recognition, pp. 558–567 (2019)
16. Hegselmann, S., Buendia, A., Lang, H., Agrawal, M., Jiang, X., Sontag, D.: TabLLM: few-shot classification of tabular data with large language models. In: International Conference on Artificial Intelligence and Statistics, pp. 5549–5581. PMLR (2023)

17. Jia, C., et al.: Scaling up visual and vision-language representation learning with noisy text supervision. In: International Conference on Machine Learning, pp. 4904–4916. PMLR (2021)

18. Kirk, H.R., Vidgen, B., Röttger, P., Hale, S.A.: Personalisation within bounds: a risk taxonomy and policy framework for the alignment of large language models with personalised feedback. arXiv preprint arXiv:2303.05453 (2023)

19. Kline, A., et al.: Multimodal machine learning in precision health: a scoping review. npj Digit. Med. **5**(1), 171 (2022)

20. Lester, B., Al-Rfou, R., Constant, N.: The power of scale for parameter-efficient prompt tuning. In: Proceedings of the 2021 Conference on Empirical Methods in Natural Language Processing, pp. 3045–3059 (2021). https://doi.org/10.18653/v1/2021.emnlp-main.243

21. Li, J., Li, D., Savarese, S., Hoi, S.: BLIP-2: bootstrapping language-image pre-training with frozen image encoders and large language models. arXiv preprint arXiv:2301.12597 (2023)

22. Lu, J., Clark, C., Zellers, R., Mottaghi, R., Kembhavi, A.: Unified-IO: a unified model for vision, language, and multi-modal tasks. arXiv preprint arXiv:2206.08916 (2022)

23. Moor, M., et al.: Foundation models for generalist medical artificial intelligence. Nature **616**(7956), 259–265 (2023)

24. OpenAI: GPT-4 technical report. arXiv preprint arXiv:2303.08774 (2023)

25. Radford, A., et al.: Learning transferable visual models from natural language supervision. In: International Conference on Machine Learning, pp. 8748–8763. PMLR (2021)

26. Recht, B., Roelofs, R., Schmidt, L., Shankar, V.: Do CIFAR-10 classifiers generalize to CIFAR-10? arXiv preprint arXiv:1806.00451 (2018)

27. Sakornsakolpat, P., et al.: Genetic landscape of chronic obstructive pulmonary disease identifies heterogeneous cell-type and phenotype associations. Nat. Genet. **51**(3), 494–505 (2019)

28. Salemi, A., Mysore, S., Bendersky, M., Zamani, H.: LaMP: when large language models meet personalization. arXiv preprint arXiv:2304.11406 (2023)

29. Shrine, N., et al.: New genetic signals for lung function highlight pathways and chronic obstructive pulmonary disease associations across multiple ancestries. Nat. Genet. **51**(3), 481–493 (2019)

30. Singhal, K., et al.: Large language models encode clinical knowledge. arXiv preprint arXiv:2212.13138 (2022)

31. Singhal, K., et al.: Towards expert-level medical question answering with large language models. arXiv preprint arXiv:2212.13138 (2022)

32. Steinberg, E., Jung, K., Fries, J.A., Corbin, C.K., Pfohl, S.R., Shah, N.H.: Language models are an effective representation learning technique for electronic health record data. J. Biomed. Inform. **113**, 103637 (2021)

33. Vestbo, J., et al.: Global strategy for the diagnosis, management, and prevention of chronic obstructive pulmonary disease. Am. J. Respir. Crit. Care Med. **187**(4), 347–365 (2013)

34. Vokinger, K.N., Feuerriegel, S., Kesselheim, A.S.: Mitigating bias in machine learning for medicine. Commun. Med. **1**(1), 25 (2021)

35. Wang, Y., et al.: Preserving in-context learning ability in large language model fine-tuning. arXiv preprint arXiv:2211.00635 (2022)

36. Wei, J., et al.: Emergent abilities of large language models. arXiv preprint arXiv:2206.07682 (2022)

37. Yang, K.D., et al.: Multi-domain translation between single-cell imaging and sequencing data using autoencoders. Nat. Commun. **12**(1), 31 (2021)
38. Yang, X., et al.: A large language model for electronic health records. npj Digit. Med. **5**(1), 194 (2022)
39. Yu, J., Wang, Z., Vasudevan, V., Yeung, L., Seyedhosseini, M., Wu, Y.: CoCa: contrastive captioners are image-text foundation models. arXiv preprint arXiv:2205.01917 (2022)
40. Zhou, H.Y., Chen, X., Zhang, Y., Luo, R., Wang, L., Yu, Y.: Generalized radiograph representation learning via cross-supervision between images and free-text radiology reports. Nat. Mach. Intell. **4**(1), 32–40 (2022)

# Speed-of-Sound Mapping for Pulse-Echo Ultrasound Raw Data Using Linked-Autoencoders

Farnaz Khun Jush[1]([⊠])(iD), Peter M. Dueppenbecker[2], and Andreas Maier[1](iD)

[1] Pattern Recognition Lab, Friedrich-Alexander-University, Erlangen, Germany
{farnaz.khun.jush,andreas.maier}@fau.de
[2] Technology Excellence, Siemens Healthcare GmbH, Erlangen, Germany
peter.dueppenbecker@siemens-healthineers.com

**Abstract.** Recent studies showed the possibility of extracting SoS information from pulse-echo ultrasound raw data (a.k.a. RF data) using deep neural networks that are fully trained on simulated data. These methods take sensor domain data, i.e., RF data, as input and train a network in an end-to-end fashion to learn the implicit mapping between the RF data domain and the SoS domain. However, such networks are prone to overfitting to simulated data which results in poor performance and instability when tested on measured data. We propose a novel method for SoS mapping employing learned representations from two linked autoencoders. We test our approach on simulated and measured data acquired from human breast mimicking phantoms. We show that SoS mapping is possible using the learned representations by linked autoencoders. The proposed method has a Mean Absolute Percentage Error (MAPE) of 2.39% on the simulated data. On the measured data, the predictions of the proposed method are close to the expected values (MAPE of 1.1%). Compared to an end-to-end trained network, the proposed method shows higher stability and reproducibility.

**Keywords:** Convolutional Autoencoder · Representation Learning · Speed-of-sound Mapping

## 1 Introduction

B-mode imaging is a qualitative approach and its outcome is dependent on the operator's expertise. Quantitative values, e.g., speed-of-sound (SoS) in tissue, can provide additional information about tissue properties. In particular, SoS is proven to be useful for differentiating tissue types in breast cancer screening [23, 24, 26]. Model-based solutions are proposed to reconstruct SoS from ultrasound pulse-echo data [25, 27, 28]. However, in the pulse-echo setup, model-based SoS reconstruction is non-trivial and such approaches require carefully chosen regularization and optimization methods, prior knowledge, and complex fine-tuning [31]. Thus, to the best of our knowledge, currently, there is no gold-standard method to reconstruct SoS.

© The Author(s), under exclusive license to Springer Nature Switzerland AG 2024
A. K. Maier et al. (Eds.): ML4MHD 2023, LNCS 14315, pp. 103–114, 2024.
https://doi.org/10.1007/978-3-031-47679-2_8

During data acquisition, the sensor encodes an intermediate representation of the object under examination in the sensor domain. The reconstruction then is performed by inversion of the corresponding encoding function [32]. However, the exact inverse function is not available a priori, thus, reconstruction problems need to approximate the function. Recently, deep neural networks are vastly being used to solve reconstruction problems. Opposed to the analytical and optimization methods where the inverse function is approximated in multiple stages of signal processing and/or optimization steps, in deep learning approaches, the network tries to solve the problem by learning the corresponding mapping between the sensor domain and reconstruction domain [32]. Therefore, during the training, a low-dimensional representation of the data in both domains is implicitly learned. This concept was first proposed in [32], a.k.a. AUTOMAP, to perform a robust reconstruction of multiple sensor-domain data. The idea is derived from domain transfer approaches, yet, no mechanism is implemented to guarantee the robustness of the solutions found by such black-box networks. Consequently, these methods are proved to be unstable, especially when the test data has perturbations or structural differences compared to training data [1].

Similar techniques are employed for SoS reconstruction from ultrasound echo data. [5, 6, 10, 12–14, 21] investigated encoder-decoder networks with multiple or single steering angles for SoS reconstruction. In these studies, an encoder-decoder network takes sensor domain data as input and directly reconstructs the SoS map in the output. Essentially, the network implicitly learns to map low-dimensional representation from the sensor data domain and SoS domain. Since there is no known gold standard method to create SoS GT from measured pulse-echo ultrasound data, all the investigated methods rely on simulated data. As such, the transfer of these methods to clinical setups is challenging and their robustness is still under debate [5, 12]. These methods are prone to overfitting the distribution of the simulated data and thus perform unsatisfactorily when tested on real data [12].

In this study, we propose a novel approach for SoS mapping from a single plane-wave acquisition. Instead of the end-to-end encoder-decoder approaches previously proposed, where an implicit mapping between the sensor domain and the SoS domain was learned, following the known operator paradigm [19], we propose a method to break the problem into two steps: In the training phase, firstly, we encode the sensor domain and the SoS domain data in an intermediate low-dimensional representation using two linked autoencoders; secondly, we find a mapping between the two representations. For inference, without any further training, parts of the autoencoders are being joined to create a network that takes the RF data as input and returns the SoS map in the output. An overview is demonstrated in Fig. 1. We then compare the proposed method with a baseline encoder-decoder network both on simulated and measured data acquired from human breast mimicking phantom.

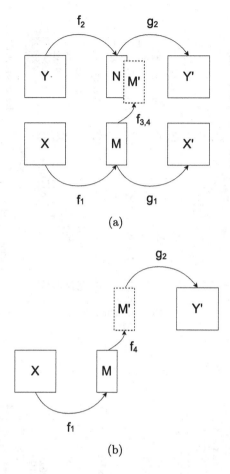

**Fig. 1.** Overview: $X$ being RF domain, $Y$ being SoS domain, $f$ encoder and $g$ decoder (a): Training: two domains are encoded to an intermediate low-dimensional representation by training two linked autoencoders jointly: $X \rightarrow f_1(X) = M \rightarrow g_1(f_1(X)) = X' \approx X$ and $Y \rightarrow f_2(Y) = N \rightarrow g_2(f_2(Y)) = Y' \approx Y$ ; plus, a mapping is performed between two representations during the training $(M \rightarrow f_3(M) = M' \approx N)$. By freezing other layers, a final fine-tuning training step is performed $(M \rightarrow f_4(M) = M' \approx N)$; (b): Inference: without further training, two steps are joined to create a network that maps the RF domain to the SoS domain: $X \rightarrow f_1(X) = M \rightarrow f_4(f_1(X)) = M' \rightarrow g_2(f_4(f_1(X))) = Y'$.

## 2   Methods

### 2.1   Network Architecture, Training

Autoencoders [2,3,18] are vastly being used to learn low-dimensional latent representations. An autoencoder maps its input to itself utilizing an intermediate

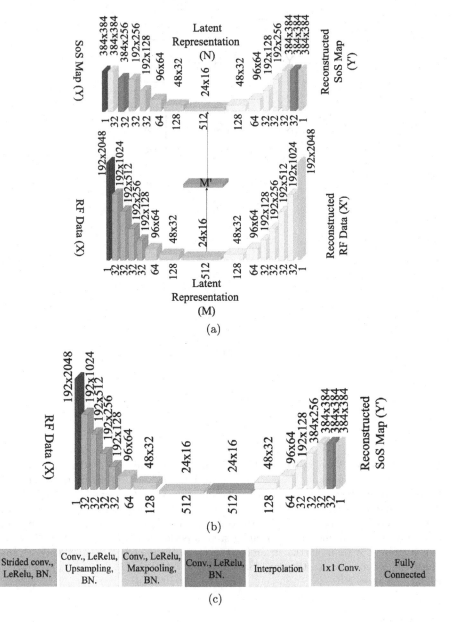

**Fig. 2. Network Architecture, Training:** (a): Linked Autoencoders: two convolutional autoencoders connected via their latent spaces that are trained jointly, Operations in each layer are color-coded. (b): **Network Architecture, Inference (AutoSpeed):** the encoding path of the trained RF Autoencoder and the decoding path of the trained SoS are joined via the trained FCL. No further training is required to employ AutoSpeed. (c): layers architecture.

representation, the so-called latent space. Autoencoders thus learn to map input data to the latent space and latent space data back to the input domain [4,30]. Hence, to learn the efficient representation from two domains, i.e., sensor domain (representing RF data) and SoS domain, autoencoders can be employed. However, since autoencoders often introduce redundancy and each feature is global [20], in order to discover localized features often convolutional autoencoders are used [4]. Convolutional autoencoders combine local convolution connections with autoencoders, thus, preserving spatial locality [4]. As such, two linked convolutional autoencoders are trained jointly.

**Linked Autoencoders.** Two convolutional autoencoders that are connected via their latent spaces are trained to extract robust features of RF data and SoS maps. During training efficient representations of the SoS domain and RF domain are encoded in the latent spaces of the autoencoders. However, these representations can have different interpretations. To bridge the gap between the aforementioned representations, they are connected via a fully connected layer (FCL) that is trained simultaneously with two autoencoders. This way, the autoencoders are optimized in a manner that the latent spaces of two networks indicate the closest possible representations. Figure 2(a) demonstrates the model architecture.

The autoencoders take the input vectors of RF and SoS domain as $x$ and $y$, respectively, and map them to the hidden representations $m$ and $n$, where, $f_{1,2}$, are the encoders with convolution and activation layers. The encoded representations, $m$ and $n$, are then used to reconstruct $x'$ and $y'$, where $g_{1,2}$ are the decoders. Each training $x^{(i)}$ and $y^{(i)}$ is thus mapped to a corresponding $m^{(i)}$ and $n^{(i)}$ and reconstructs $x'^{(i)}$ and $y'^{(i)}$ Fig. 1. Simultaneously, the latent spaces are being optimized to match: $m$ is mapped to $m'$ via an FCL, $m' = f_3(m)$. During the training $m', n$ are being optimized in the loss function to match closely, where $m' = f_3(f_1(x))$ and $n = f_2(y)$ Fig. 1. The following cost function is optimized:

$$
\begin{aligned}
J_{LAE} &= \frac{1}{n} \sum_{i=1}^{N} \left[ L(x^{(i)}, x'^{(i)}) + L(y^{(i)}, y'^{(i)}) + L(m'^{(i)}, n^{(i)}) \right] \\
&= \frac{1}{n} \sum_{i=1}^{N} \left[ L(x^{(i)}, g_1(f_1(x^{(i)}))) + L(y^{(i)}, g_2(f_2(y^{(i)}))) + L(f_3(f_1(x^{(i)})), f_2(y^{(i)})) \right]
\end{aligned}
\tag{1}
$$

where L is the loss function, here the Mean Squared Error (MSE), $L(x, x') = ||x - x'||^2$, is used. Note that for simplification, vector representation is used in the text but Fig. 2 shows matrix representation.

After convergence of the linked autoencoders, to fine-tune the FCL, all other layers are frozen and the training continues only on the FCL, thus the following cost function is optimized:

$$J_{FCL} = \frac{1}{n} \sum_{i=1}^{N} L(n, m') = \frac{1}{n} \sum_{i=1}^{N} L(n, f_4(m)) \qquad (2)$$

## 2.2  Network Architecture, Inference

For the inference, we propose a network that henceforth will be referred to as AutoSpeed. AutoSpeed is an encoder-decoder network that its encoder is detached from the trained RF autoencoder and its decoder is detached from the trained SoS autoencoder. Extracted encoder and decoder paths are connected via the FCL that was trained jointly with the autoencoders. Note that there is no retraining step required to employ the AutoSpeed, the layers are simply taken from the trained linked networks as modules.

# 3  Results

For SoS reconstruction, acquiring sufficient measured data is challenging, thus, using simulated data for training is a common practice [5,6,10,12–14,21,31]. K-Wave toolbox [29] (Version 1.3) is used for the simulation of training data. The LightABVS system [9,13], an in-house digital ultrasound prototype system that consists of a linear probe with 192 active channels, a pitch of $200\,\mu$m, and a center frequency of 5 MHz is used for data acquisition. The size of the medium is considered to be $3.8 \times 7.6$ cm in depth and lateral direction ($1536 \times 3072$ grid points). The probe head is placed above the central section of the medium. A single plane-wave with zero degrees is used [6,12,13]. The simulation setup for training data generation is a joint set of datasets proposed by [5,12], further details can be found [12].

## 3.1  Training, Linked Autoencoder

The linked autoencoder is trained for 200 epochs (SGD optimizer, batch size of 8). The training dataset had 6000 cases (4800 training, 1200 validation) and the test dataset had 150 cases based on [5,12,13].

**RF Autoencoder.** Over 10 training runs, the RF autoencoder converges to an average Root Mean Squared Error (RMSE) of $6.06 \pm 0.31$ (SoS $\pm$ SD where SD is the standard deviation) and Mean Absolute Error (MAE) of $3.94 \pm 0.29$, where the input RF data is in the range $[-1024, 1024]$. It is noteworthy that during training experiments we observed that normalization hinders the convergence of RF Autoencoder, thus, the data is not normalized.

**SoS Autoencoder.** The SoS autoencoder converges to RMSE of 7.89±3.23 m/s and MAE of 6.68 ± 3.03 m/s, where the input range is [1300, 1700] m/s.

**FCL.** The FCL-layer is trained for 150 epochs using the Adam optimizer, where it converges to RMSE of 0.68 ± 0.28 and MAE of 0.55 ± 0.19 over 10 training runs, where the output of mid-layers is in the range [−15, 30].

### 3.2  Inference, Simulated Data

On the test dataset, AutoSpeed has an average RMSE of 47.98 ± 4.15 m/s, MAE of 37.26 ± 3.56 m/s and MAPE of 2.39 ± 0.22% over 10 training runs.

We set up an end-to-end trained encoder-decoder network based on [12] and compared the results of AutoSpeed with this network. Hereafter, we will refer to the baseline network as En-De-Net. The architecture of En-De-Net is exactly the same as in Fig. 2(c), only the FCL is removed. The En-De-Net converges to RMSE of 23.64 ± 0.7 m/s, MAE 17.32 ± 0.7 m/s, and MAPE of 1.11 ± 0.05%. The error ranges of both networks are in the typical range of SoS errors (1–2%) [5,11,12,21]. However, on the simulated data, the En-De-Net has a lower error rate. Nevertheless, [15,22] showed that the presence of breast lesions results in SoS contrast in comparison with the background tissue, e.g., this contrast is in the range of [14–118] m/s and [7–41] m/s for malignant and benign lesions, respectively. Thus, theoretically, the predicted values are relevant for clinical use cases.

### 3.3  Inference, Measured Data

We performed an experiment with measured data from CIRS multi-modality breast mimicking phantom to demonstrate the stability and reproducibility of AutoSpeed predictions compared to En-De-Net when tested on real data acquired from the same field of view for multiple frames. We acquired 200 frames when the probe head and phantom is mechanically fixed. The expectation is that the networks predict consistent SoS values inside the inclusion and in the background for similar frames. Additionally, we expect that the SoS values inside the inclusion have low SD.

Figure 3 shows 4 cases of the aforementioned dataset. AutoSpeed predicted SoS values in the range 1535±6 m/s and 1561±11 m/s in the background region and inside the inclusion area, respectively, where the corresponding expected values are 1520 ± 10 m/s and 1580 ± 20 m/s. Whereas En-De-Net has predicted SoS range 1527±19 m/s in the background and 1545±45 m/s inside the inclusion. Although both networks follow the geometry in the corresponding b-mode images and could find the inclusion and the skin layer and background margin correctly, AutoSpeed shows more consistency. In Fig. 3, Frame 1 green arrows in the En-De-Net prediction image show the inconsistent regions that appear differently from frame to frame, e.g., on the left side of the image, the SoS values are inverted compared to the background (lower to higher and back to lower) from one frame to another frame. On the right side of the image, there is a region detected with SoS contrast, but the margin and the SoS values in the corresponding region vary. The same can be observed in the inclusion area in the middle. Whereas, the predictions of the AutoSpeed network are consistent throughout all the frames.

Figure 4 compares the mean SoS values inside the inclusion and in the background as well as their corresponding SD. Based on Fig. 4(a) and (b), AutoSpeed has highly consistent predictions both inside the inclusion and in the background in consecutive frames. Additionally, Fig. 4(c) and (d) show that the SoS values in each frame inside the inclusion and in the background have consistent uniformity for AutoSpeed compared to En-De-Net. Thus, AutoSpeed can extract more stable features compared to the En-De-Net which performs an end-to-end mapping and thus lower error rates on the simulated data do not necessarily translate to the measured data.

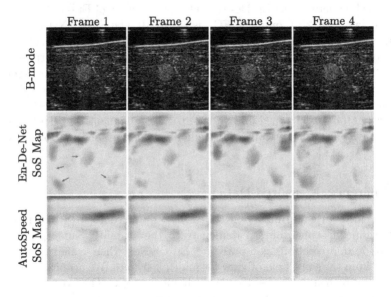

**Fig. 3.** AutoSpeed vs. En-De-Net: Predicted SoS maps by AutoSpeed are more consistent for the same field of view. (Color figure online)

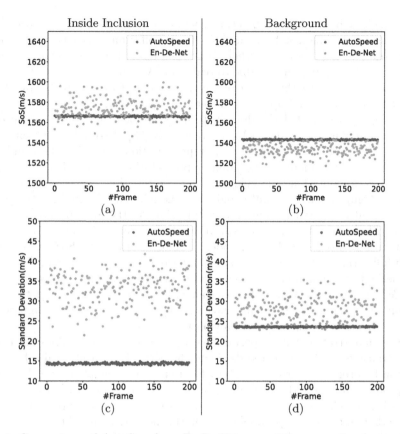

**Fig. 4.** Comparison of AutoSpeed vs. En-De-Net, over 200 consecutive frames from the same field of view: the average predicted SoS values inside the inclusion **(a)**: and in the background **(b)**: The SD of the predictions inside the inclusion **(c)**: and in the background **(d)**: The predicted SoS values by AutoSpeed are more consistent through all the frames compared to En-De-Net.

## 4    Discussion and Conclusion

SoS reconstruction for pulse-echo ultrasound can be advantageous in clinical studies because it employs the available data acquisition setups used for B-mode imaging and provides quantitative measures. Yet, it is still in its infancy stage and no accepted gold-standard method is available. Analytical and optimization-based methods require prior and carefully chosen regularization parameters and the proposed methods are often either not stable and/or not feasible for real-time applications. In recent years, deep learning techniques are widely used to solve inverse problems that perform on par or even in some cases outperform model-based methods. Additionally, they move the computational burden to the training phase, thus, in inference, they can perform real-time. But they need training data often alongside their labels or GT maps. Hence, the lack of a gold standard method for SoS reconstruction poses a challenge to developing deep learning techniques. Simulation toolboxes offer an alternative solution to create training data. However, there is no guarantee that the networks trained on simulated data are transferable to real data. As a result, incorporating prior knowledge can increase the chance of success of such networks in real data setups.

We proposed a novel approach inspired by the known parameter paradigm [16,17,19], we hardcoded the domain transfer problem in a dual autoencoder approach, similar to the idea behind Cycle-GAN [33]. Two linked autoencoders are trained jointly to extract efficient representations from RF data and SoS maps and an FCL mapped the latent representation of the RF data domain to the SoS domain. There is evidence that the functions learned by networks can be decomposed into modules and those modules can be used in other tasks even without any further training [7,8,16]. Thus, in the inference, an encoder-decoder-like architecture is proposed in which the encoder is detached from the RF data autoencoder and the decoder is detached from the SoS autoencoder (both fully trained) and two paths are connected via a trained FCL. We tested the method on simulated and measured data and compared the results with an encoder-decoder network that is trained end-to-end. We showed that SoS mapping is possible by employing such a setup and is more stable compared to the end-to-end mapping solution previously proposed.

We demonstrated that outperforming on the simulated data does not necessarily translate to the measured data and the networks that are trained end-to-end can be prone to overfitting to the distribution of simulated data. Whereas, our proposed method that employs the learned representations from autoencoders is more stable, can extract efficient features, and outperforms the end-to-end method in terms of reproducibility. On the measured data, AutoSpeed could detect the inclusions and correct margins, and the predicted SoS maps are close to the expected range. The downside of this method compared to the simple encoder-decoder network is that due to the usage of two autoencoders, the number of parameters and time of training are twice. Nevertheless, due to the similar architecture in the inference, the time does not change. The initial results are highly encouraging but further research is required to transfer and prove the efficiency of such methods in clinical setups. Nevertheless, this approach can have more generalized use-cases and can potentially replace the end-to-end encoder-decoder networks that are currently being used for reconstruction purposes.

## Disclaimer

The information in this paper is based on research results that are not commercially available.

**Acknowledgments.** We thank Prof. Michael Golatta and the university hospital of Heidelberg for providing the Tomosynthesis dataset.

# References

1. Antun, V., Renna, F., Poon, C., Adcock, B., Hansen, A.C.: On instabilities of deep learning in image reconstruction and the potential costs of AI. Proc. Natl. Acad. Sci. **117**(48), 30088–30095 (2020)
2. Bengio, Y.: Learning Deep Architectures for AI. Now Publishers Inc. (2009)
3. Bengio, Y., Courville, A., Vincent, P.: Representation learning: a review and new perspectives. IEEE Trans. Pattern Anal. Mach. Intell. **35**(8), 1798–1828 (2013)
4. Chen, M., Shi, X., Zhang, Y., Wu, D., Guizani, M.: Deep features learning for medical image analysis with convolutional autoencoder neural network. IEEE Trans. Big Data **7**, 750–758 (2017)
5. Feigin, M., Freedman, D., Anthony, B.W.: A deep learning framework for single-sided sound speed inversion in medical ultrasound. IEEE Trans. Biomed. Eng. **67**(4), 1142–1151 (2019)
6. Feigin, M., Zwecker, M., Freedman, D., Anthony, B.W.: Detecting muscle activation using ultrasound speed of sound inversion with deep learning. In: 2020 42nd Annual International Conference of the IEEE Engineering in Medicine & Biology Society (EMBC), pp. 2092–2095. IEEE (2020)
7. Fu, W., Breininger, K., Schaffert, R., Ravikumar, N., Maier, A.: A divide-and-conquer approach towards understanding deep networks. In: Shen, D., et al. (ed.) Medical Image Computing and Computer Assisted Intervention, MICCAI 2019. LNCS, vol. 11764, pp. 183–191. Springer, Cham (2019). https://doi.org/10.1007/978-3-030-32239-7_21
8. Fu, W., Husvogt, L., Ploner, S., Fujimoto, J.G., Maier, A.: Modularization of deep networks allows cross-modality reuse. In: Bildverarbeitung für die Medizin 2020. I, pp. 274–279. Springer, Wiesbaden (2020). https://doi.org/10.1007/978-3-658-29267-6_61
9. Hager, P.A., Khun Jush, F., Biele, M., Düppenbecker, P.M., Schmidt, O., Benini, L.: LightABVS: a digital ultrasound transducer for multi-modality automated breast volume scanning. In: 2019 IEEE International Ultrasonics Symposium (IUS) (2019)
10. Heller, M., Schmitz, G.: Deep learning-based speed-of-sound reconstruction for single-sided pulse-echo ultrasound using a coherency measure as input feature. In: 2021 IEEE International Ultrasonics Symposium (IUS), pp. 1–4. IEEE (2021)
11. Hill, C.R., Bamber, J.C., ter Haar, G.R.: Physical Principles of Medical Ultrasonics (2004)
12. Khun Jush, F., Biele, M., Dueppenbecker, P.M., Maier, A.: Deep learning for ultrasound speed-of-sound reconstruction: impacts of training data diversity on stability and robustness. MELBA J. Mach. Learn. Biomed. Imaging **2**, 202–236 (2023)
13. Khun Jush, F., Biele, M., Dueppenbecker, P.M., Schmidt, O., Maier, A.: DNN-based speed-of-sound reconstruction for automated breast ultrasound. In: 2020 IEEE International Ultrasonics Symposium (IUS), pp. 1–7. IEEE (2020)
14. Khun Jush, F., Dueppenbecker, P.M., Maier, A.: Data-driven speed-of-sound reconstruction for medical ultrasound: impacts of training data format and imperfections on convergence. In: Papież, B.W., Yaqub, M., Jiao, J., Namburete, A.I.L., Noble, J.A. (eds.) MIUA 2021. LNCS, vol. 12722, pp. 140–150. Springer, Cham (2021). https://doi.org/10.1007/978-3-030-80432-9_11
15. Li, C., Duric, N., Littrup, P., Huang, L.: In vivo breast sound-speed imaging with ultrasound tomography. Ultrasound Med. Biol. **35**(10), 1615–1628 (2009)

16. Maier, A., Köstler, H., Heisig, M., Krauss, P., Yang, S.H.: Known operator learning and hybrid machine learning in medical imaging - a review of the past, the present, and the future. Prog. Biomed. Eng. **4**, 022002 (2022)

17. Maier, A., et al.: Precision learning: towards use of known operators in neural networks. In: 2018 24th International Conference on Pattern Recognition (ICPR), pp. 183–188. IEEE (2018)

18. Maier, A., Syben, C., Lasser, T., Riess, C.: A gentle introduction to deep learning in medical image processing. Z. Med. Phys. **29**(2), 86–101 (2019)

19. Maier, A.K., et al.: Learning with known operators reduces maximum error bounds. Nat. Mach. Intell. **1**(8), 373–380 (2019)

20. Masci, J., Meier, U., Cireşan, D., Schmidhuber, J.: Stacked convolutional auto-encoders for hierarchical feature extraction. In: Honkela, T., Duch, W., Girolami, M., Kaski, S. (eds.) ICANN 2011. LNCS, vol. 6791, pp. 52–59. Springer, Heidelberg (2011). https://doi.org/10.1007/978-3-642-21735-7_7

21. Oh, S.H., Kim, M.-G., Kim, Y., Kwon, H., Bae, H.-M.: A neural framework for multi-variable lesion quantification through b-mode style transfer. In: de Bruijne, M., et al. (eds.) MICCAI 2021. LNCS, vol. 12906, pp. 222–231. Springer, Cham (2021). https://doi.org/10.1007/978-3-030-87231-1_22

22. Ruby, L., et al.: Breast cancer assessment with pulse-echo speed of sound ultra-sound from intrinsic tissue reflections: proof-of-concept. Invest. Radiol. **54**(7), 419–427 (2019)

23. Sak, M., et al.: Using speed of sound imaging to characterize breast density. Ultra-sound Med. Biol. **43**(1), 91–103 (2017)

24. Sanabria, S.J., et al.: Breast-density assessment with hand-held ultrasound: a novel biomarker to assess breast cancer risk and to tailor screening? Eur. Radiol. **28**(8), 3165–3175 (2018)

25. Sanabria, S.J., Rominger, M.B., Goksel, O.: Speed-of-sound imaging based on reflector delineation. IEEE Trans. Biomed. Eng. **66**(7), 1949–1962 (2018)

26. Schreiman, J., Gisvold, J., Greenleaf, J.F., Bahn, R.: Ultrasound transmission computed tomography of the breast. Radiology **150**(2), 523–530 (1984)

27. Stähli, P., Frenz, M., Jaeger, M.: Bayesian approach for a robust speed-of-sound reconstruction using pulse-echo ultrasound. IEEE Trans. Med. Imaging **40**(2), 457–467 (2020)

28. Stähli, P., Kuriakose, M., Frenz, M., Jaeger, M.: Improved forward model for quantitative pulse-echo speed-of-sound imaging. Ultrasonics **108**, 106168 (2020)

29. Treeby, B.E., Cox, B.T.: k-Wave: MATLAB toolbox for the simulation and reconstruction of photoacoustic wave fields. J. Biomed. Opt. **15**(2), 021314 (2010)

30. Vincent, P., Larochelle, H., Bengio, Y., Manzagol, P.A.: Extracting and composing robust features with denoising autoencoders. In: Proceedings of the 25th International Conference on Machine Learning, pp. 1096–1103 (2008)

31. Vishnevskiy, V., Sanabria, S.J., Goksel, O.: Image reconstruction via variational network for real-time hand-held sound-speed imaging. In: Knoll, F., Maier, A., Rueckert, D. (eds.) MLMIR 2018. LNCS, vol. 11074, pp. 120–128. Springer, Cham (2018). https://doi.org/10.1007/978-3-030-00129-2_14

32. Zhu, B., Liu, J.Z., Cauley, S.F., Rosen, B.R., Rosen, M.S.: Image reconstruction by domain-transform manifold learning. Nature **555**(7697), 487–492 (2018)

33. Zhu, J.Y., Park, T., Isola, P., Efros, A.A.: Unpaired image-to-image translation using cycle-consistent adversarial networks. In: Proceedings of the IEEE International Conference on Computer Vision, pp. 2223–2232 (2017)

# HOOREX: Higher Order Optimizers for 3D Recovery from X-Ray Images

Karthik Shetty[1,2(✉)], Annette Birkhold[2], Bernhard Egger[1],
Srikrishna Jaganathan[1,2], Norbert Strobel[2,3], Markus Kowarschik[2],
and Andreas Maier[1]

[1] Friedrich-Alexander Universität Erlangen-Nürnberg, Erlangen, Germany
`karthik.shetty@fau.de`
[2] Siemens Healthcare GmbH, Erlangen, Germany
[3] University of Applied Sciences Würzburg-Schweinfurt, Würzburg, Germany

**Abstract.** We propose a method to address the challenge of generating a 3D digital twin of a patient during an X-ray guided medical procedure from a single 2D X-ray projection image, a problem that is inherently ill-posed. To tackle this issue, we aim to infer the parameters of Bones, Organs and Skin Shape (BOSS) model, a deformable human shape and pose model. There are currently two main approaches for model-based estimation. Optimization-based methods try to iteratively fit a body model to 2D measurements, they produce accurate 2D alignments but are slow and sensitive to initialization. On the other hand, regression-based methods use neural networks to estimate the model parameters directly, resulting in faster predictions but often with misalignments. Our approach combines the benefits of both techniques by implementing a fully differentiable paradigm through the use of higher-order optimizers that only require the Jacobian, which can be determined implicitly. The network was trained on synthetic CT and real CBCT image data, ensuring view independence. We demonstrate the potential clinical applicability of our method by validating it on multiple datasets covering diverse anatomical regions, and achieving an error of 27.98 mm.

## 1 Introduction

In an interventional imaging setting, digital twins of patients and procedures have the potential to optimize various clinical tasks and workflow steps or support radiation safety [16]. However, for most tasks, a patient model must accurately represent the shape and pose of the actual patient during the intervention. Typically, only demographic information, such as age, weight, height and gender of the patient is available prior to the procedure to generate a patient-specific model. However, generating a patient-specific model directly from the first X-ray images obtained during a procedure could significantly improve the patient model, as it would, besides patient shape, allow to estimate position and pose of the patient on the interventional table [24].

© The Author(s), under exclusive license to Springer Nature Switzerland AG 2024
A. K. Maier et al. (Eds.): ML4MHD 2023, LNCS 14315, pp. 115–124, 2024.
https://doi.org/10.1007/978-3-031-47679-2_9

Over the years, there has been extensive research in estimating human pose and shape for body, face, or hand from single images [14,22,26]. While early methods predicted landmarks or joints, recent techniques directly regress the parameters of a parametric model such as the Skinned Multi-Person Linear model (SMPL) [12] for human bodies. However, applying these concepts to X-ray imaging was challenging due to limited data availability and the absence of parametric models of the skeleton and other organs. The recent development of skeleton models such as OSSO [6] and BOSS [19] has enabled us to use these methods in the medical field. Previous approaches to generate shape and pose models in the medical field relied on Statistical Shape Models (SSM) or Statistical Shape Intensity Models (SSIM) for extremely specific bone structures or organs [1,10]. These models often relied on global optimizers, but had limitations such as being based on visual cues and only applicable to a small portion of the image, as well as not being view-independent. There are generally two major approaches to solving this problem: image similarity metrics and feature descriptors. In the presence of SSIMs, image similarity techniques can be used, where a synthetically generated intensity image is iteratively optimized with respect to the real image based on a relevant loss metric. Feature-based approaches use an intermediate process such as landmarks or feature descriptors for the optimization process. Therefore, most recent works make use of deep learning, either directly or indirectly, to determine the features used for the model generation process. 3D Knee bone model generation from bi-planar X-ray images was demonstrated by training on synthetic data and using style transfer for domain adaptation [5]. Volumetric model generation from single or multiple images was proposed as a method for generating surrogate CT images [18,25].

As previously stated, model-based estimation can be tackled using either Optimization-based methods or regression-based methods, each with their own limitations. However, analytical solvers [11,20] offer an alternative solution to this problem by combining both approaches and restructuring the problem as a closed-form solution. Nevertheless, the main drawback of these methods is often related to the structure of the training data, which requires ground-truth model parameters or aligned keypoints within the kinematic chain of the skeleton, making the creation of suitable training data cumbersome. Our proposed solution is to leverage the simpler regression method as prior knowledge learned by the network and iteratively optimize the re-projection error from its predictions in a differentiable manner to improve the 2D alignment. To this end, we propose an adaptive approach to train the neural network for skeleton model generation by fusing a regression-based method with an optimization-based method.

## 2  Methods

Our proposed framework predicts a 3D mesh model of the skeleton from a single projection image. We make use of the BOSS [19] model as the parametric bone model and the Human Mesh Recovery (HMR) [4,9] framework as the regression network, as illustrated in Fig. 1. We present a brief overview of the shape model and regression network employed, followed by our approach to obtaining absolute depth, which addresses warping effects. Finally, we discuss how we employ higher-order optimizers and integrate all components of our framework.

## 2.1   BOSS Model

The skeleton of the BOSS [19] model, a derivative of the SMPL [12] model, is utilized as the skeletal model and offers a differentiable function $\mathcal{M}(\theta, \beta)$ that generates a mesh $M \in \mathbb{R}^{N \times 3}$ with $N = 65,617$ vertices. The shape parameters $\beta$ are expressed by a low-dimensional principal component, mapping the linear basis $\mathbf{B}$ from $\mathbb{R}^{|\beta|} \mapsto \mathbb{R}^{N \times 3}$. This represents the offsets from the average mesh $\bar{x}_m$ as $x = \bar{x}_m + \beta \mathbf{B}$. The pose $\theta$ of the model is determined by a kinematic chain that incorporates a set of relative rotation vectors $\theta = [\theta_1, \ldots, \theta_K] \in \mathbb{R}^{K \times 3}$, consisting of $K = 63$ joints represented using axis-angle rotations. In this paper, we disregard the skin and organ meshes produced by the complete BOSS model and use only the bone model. In this study, we focus on specific vertices $\mathbf{X}_{3D} \subset M$ on the surface of the mesh, totaling $N_j = 112$, as landmarks of interest which we represent as $\mathcal{M}_l$.

## 2.2   Regression Network

Our regression model utilizes a deep neural network, with an architecture similar to that of HMR [4,9]. The only difference lies in the choice of encoder, where we opt for efficientnet-v2-s [21] over Resnet-50, as we observe faster convergence during training. The encoder serves as a feature extractor denoted by $\mathbf{F} \in \mathbb{R}^{C \times c \times c}$, with a channel dimension of $C = 272$ and height and width of $c = 9$. The input for the encoder is a cropped X-ray image $\mathbf{I} \in \mathbb{R}^{3 \times 288 \times 288}$. Following this, an iterative MultiLayer Perceptron regressor is employed to predict the model parameters $\boldsymbol{\Theta}_r = \{\theta_r, \beta_r\}$ and the virtual camera parameters $\boldsymbol{\Pi}_r = \{t_x, t_y, s\}$. Here, $t_x$ and $t_y$ are the root translations for the cropped image, and $s$ denotes the scaling factor. However, this approach proves problematic in the X-ray imaging context because the subject of interest is positioned between the source and detector. Consequently, significant perspective warping occurs [2], which cannot be effectively handled using a weak-camera model.

**Absolute Depth.** To address the aforementioned issues, we assume a calibrated camera system and employ an absolute depth estimation. This approach requires a set of 3D points and their corresponding 2D points on the image plane. Assuming that $\mathbf{X}_{3D}$ represents the network predicted root-relative 3D keypoints for model parameters $\boldsymbol{\Theta}_r$, we still need to predict the corresponding 2D landmarks represented as $\mathbf{x}_{uv}$. To accomplish this, we up-sample the encoder output $\mathbf{F}$ to a resolution of 72 pixels, and then utilize a lixel-representation [13] to predict the 2D landmarks on the x-y axis individually. In a similar manner, we also regress weights $\mathbf{w}$ which indicate whether the given landmarks exists inside the region-of-interest. We opted for the lixel-representation, which utilizes pixel-aligned lines to represent heatmaps, as it is more memory-efficient and can be easily scaled up to predict dense landmarks.

The calibrated projection matrix that accounts for the affine transformation, such as cropping and resizing, for the input image into the network is denoted by the matrix $\mathbf{K} \in \mathbb{R}^{3 \times 4}$. In an ideal perspective-camera setting, the relationship between the 3D and 2D predicted landmarks can be expressed as

$$\mathbf{K}[\mathbf{I}|\mathbf{t}](\mathbf{w} \odot \mathbf{X}_{3D})^T = (\mathbf{w} \odot \mathbf{x}_{uv})^T \tag{1}$$

under homogeneous coordinates. Here, $\mathbf{t}$ denotes the absolute offset necessary to align the 3D and 2D landmarks. This being an over-determined system in general is solved using Direct Linear Transform (DLT) in a differentiable manner through QR-decomposition [20].

### 2.3    Second Order In-the-Loop Optimization

The procedure to estimate the model parameters $\mathbf{\Theta}_r$ using the HMR model is highly non-linear and neglects the imaging system's characteristics, leading to the possibility of misaligned images. However, we can fine-tune the prediction using iterative methods within the training loop once the network has learned to perform reasonably accurate regression. We believe that since neural networks can predict 2D landmarks effectively, we can leverage them to guide the refinement of the model parameters.

Our objective is to minimize the re-projection loss between the network-predicted model parameters and the 2D landmarks estimated by the network. This residual can be expressed as

$$r(\mathbf{\Psi}) = \mathbf{K}\left(\mathcal{M}_l(\mathbf{\Theta}_r) + \mathbf{t}\right) - \mathbf{x}_{2D}, \tag{2}$$

where $\mathbf{\Psi} = \{\mathbf{\Theta}_r, \mathbf{t}\}$. To achieve this goal, we minimize a non-linear least squares problem, which can be formulated as $f(\mathbf{\Psi}) = \frac{1}{2}||r(\mathbf{\Psi})||^2$. The derivative of $f$ with respect to $r$ is expressed by the Jacobian matrix $\nabla f(\mathbf{\Psi}) = J(\mathbf{\Psi})^T r(\mathbf{\Psi})$. While gradient descent is the most straightforward method for finding the minima of this function, it can be improved using second-order methods like Newton's method, which maintains end-to-end differentiability. By solving for the equation $\nabla f(\mathbf{\Psi}) = 0$, we can update the parameters $\mathbf{\Psi}$ for each iteration. A common approach to solve this is to approximate with Taylor expansion by ignoring higher-order terms, resulting in

$$\nabla f(\mathbf{\Psi}_{n+1}) = 0 = \nabla f(\mathbf{\Psi}_n) + (\mathbf{\Psi}_{n+1} - \mathbf{\Psi}_n)\nabla^2 f(\mathbf{\Psi}_n). \tag{3}$$

Assuming that the residuals are small, the Hessian matrix $H$ can be approximated as $\nabla^2 f(\mathbf{\Psi}) = J^T J$. The update step for Newton's method can then be written as

$$\mathbf{\Psi}_{n+1} = \mathbf{\Psi}_n - (\nabla^2 f(\mathbf{\Psi}_n))^+ \nabla f(\mathbf{\Psi}_n) = \mathbf{\Psi}_n - H^+ J^T r. \tag{4}$$

Here, $H^+$ represents the inverse of the Hessian. The Levenberg-Marquardt (LM) algorithm modifies the Newton method, as shown in Eq. 4, to provide an optimal step. The updated equation is as follows

$$\boldsymbol{\Psi}_{n+1} = \boldsymbol{\Psi}_n - (H + \lambda H_{diag})^+ J^T r, \tag{5}$$

where $\lambda$ is the damping factor.

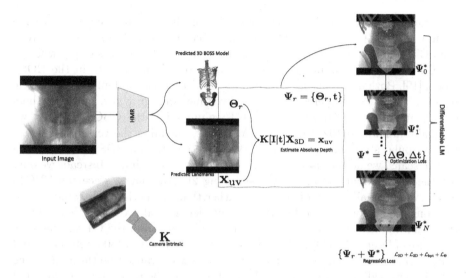

**Fig. 1.** The model generation pipeline involves the use of regression networks based on HMR for predicting model parameters $\boldsymbol{\Theta}_r$ and 2D key-points $\mathbf{x}_{uv}$ in the image space. The 3D keypoints obtained from the model parameters along with their corresponding predicted 2D landmarks allow for the estimation of the absolute depth $\mathbf{t}$ for a given camera. These parameters are then utilized as the initial values for the LM optimizer, which minimizes the re-projection error.

## 2.4   Loss Functions

Since the entire pipeline is differentiable, we train the network end-to-end. We obtain the total loss by minimizing the following equation

$$\mathcal{L} = \omega_{3D}\mathcal{L}_{3D} + \omega_{2D}\mathcal{L}_{2D} + \omega_{kpt}\mathcal{L}_{kpt} + \omega_{\Theta}\mathcal{L}_{\Theta}.$$

Here, $\mathcal{L}_{3D} = ||\mathbf{X}_{3D} - \hat{\mathbf{X}}_{3D}||_1$ minimizes the 3D keypoint loss, $\mathcal{L}_{2D} = ||\mathbf{x}_{2D} - \hat{\mathbf{x}}_{2D}||_1$ minimizes the 2D re-projection loss, $\mathcal{L}_{kpt} = ||\mathbf{x}_{uv} - \hat{\mathbf{x}}_{2D}||_1$ minimizes the 2D keypoint necessary for absolute depth prediction and LM minimization, and finally $\mathcal{L}_{\Theta} = ||\Theta - \hat{\Theta}||_2$ minimizes the BOSS model parameters. The coefficients $\omega_{3D}, \omega_{2D}, \omega_{uvw}$, and $\omega_{\Theta}$ are weighting factors applied to the corresponding loss functions. Depending on the experiment, the 2D re-projection loss can either utilize the weak camera model with network-predicted translation $\Pi$ or the full-perspective camera with the absolute depth $t$ that has been analytically solved.

## 3    Experiments and Results

### 3.1    Data

The training dataset consists of a combination of 13k X-ray projections from cone beam CT (CBCT) scans and 300k Digitally Reconstructed Radiography (DRR) from CT volumes. The CBCT data was provided by the authors of [3], whereas the CT datasets are publicly available and were also used to train the BOSS model [19]. Both datasets comprise images of the thoracic, abdominal, and pelvic regions. The BOSS model fits to the CT volumes were provided by the authors of [19] and include 306 whole-body CT volumes For the CBCT dataset, we manually annotated 102 significant landmarks, including the vertebrae, pelvis, ribs, scapula, sternum, and clavicle. While we can fit the BOSS model to the CBCT scans, we do not use the model parameters for training. Instead, we only use the 3D landmarks and its corresponding 2D landmarks, since the CBCTs only covers a small region of the body rather than the entire body. Since we do not consider the projection direction, we flip left lateral projection images to a right viewing direction. To generate synthetic images from the CT volumes, we make use of DeepDRR [23] with a focal length in the range of $(800, 1200)$ mm and a detector size of 1240 mm. We generate samples with translation throughout the volume across all axis and with random rotations in the range of $(-90, 90)°$ and $(-30, 30)°$ around LAO/RAO and CRAN/CAUD centred around the AP view respectively. Detector rotation is done implicitly during training and evaluation.

Our evaluation is conducted on 6 CBCT scans [3], 78 CT scans from the ACRIN [7] dataset, and 374 CT scans from the VerSe dataset [17]. For the CBCT scans, we evaluated our results against manually annotated landmarks. Whereas for the ACRIN dataset, we evaluated against the registered BOSS model, while for the VerSe dataset, we evaluated on the provided landmarks. As the landmarks on the VerSe dataset lie inside the spine, we registered the vertebra from the BOSS model to the VerSe segmentations and generated a linear mapping from the mesh vertices to the landmarks. This regressor was used during the final evaluation. Furthermore, volumes containing L6 or T13 vertebra are excluded from the verse dataset evaluation since the BOSS model is unable to handle them.

### 3.2    Experimental Setup

The training strategy is as follows: we pre-train the HMR model for two epochs, followed by two more epochs of pre-training with absolute depth to prevent instability during training. The reason for this is that sub-optimal 2D landmark predictions can lead to an ill-conditioned matrix used for analytically solving for depth. The final training is conducted using end-to-end LM optimization within the loop, with the loss function described in Sect. 2.4 The weights for $\omega_{3D}, \omega_{2D}, \omega_{kpt}$, and $\omega_{\Theta}$ are empirically set to 5, 5, 8, and 1, respectively. We set the damping factor $\lambda$ for the LM step to 0.1 and iterate for $n = 5$ steps. The training is performed for a total of 20 epochs on Nvidia RTX 2080S with a batch size of 16. We use Adam [8] optimizer with a learning rate of $1e^{-4}$ for pre-training and $5e^{-5}$ for the final training using PyTorch. We utilize Theseus [15] to perform the LM optimization, and it employs the AutoGrad function from PyTorch to compute the Jacobian. To evaluate our model's performance, we use standard error metrics like the Mean Per Joint Position Error (MPJPE) as used in previous related works [4, 20].

**Table 1.** To illustrate the effects of our framework, we ablate over different components used in our proposed method using the ACRIN CT dataset during both training and evaluation.

| Training | | Evalutation | | Results | |
|---|---|---|---|---|---|
| Abs. Depth | Opt. | Abs. Depth | Opt. | MPJPE$_{3D}$ (mm) | MPJPE$_{2D}$ (px) |
| ✗ | ✗ | ✗ | ✗ | 33.58 | 11.06 |
| ✓ | ✗ | ✓ | ✗ | 28.88 | 5.95 |
| ✓ | ✗ | ✓ | ✓ | 29.02 | 5.65 |
| ✓ | ✓ | ✓ | ✓ | **27.98** | **5.11** |
| ✗ | ✗ | ✗ | ✓ | 30.07 | 6.40 |
| ✓ | ✓ | ✓ | ✗ | 30.45 | 6.38 |

### 3.3   Results

As we could not identify previous studies in the field of medical imaging aiming for a 3D whole skeleton model generation from a single projection image, we use the HMR model as reference, which is widely regarded as a strong base model. To determine the significance of specific components of our method as presented in Table 1, we conducted ablation studies using the ACRIN dataset. The 3D and 2D error of the baseline method are 33.58 mm and 11.06 px, respectively, while our proposed method using absolute depth and an optimizer reduces them to 27.98 mm and 5.11 px, respectively. Table 2 summarized the outcomes of our complete approach on the different evaluated datasets. Furthermore, we present a qualitative results of our proposed method in Fig. 2. The runtime of our proposed approach takes approximately 166 ms.

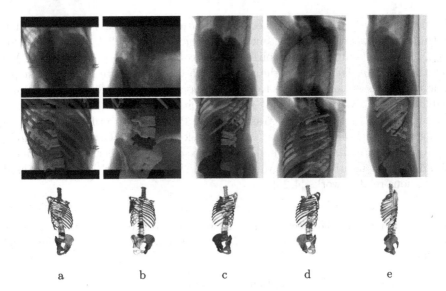

a          b          c          d          e

**Fig. 2.** The predicted 3D mesh and mesh overlay are shown in the second and third rows, respectively, following the input image in the first row. These imges were obtained from CBCT (a,b), DRRs from ACRIN (c,d), and VerSe (e).

**Table 2.** Performance assessment on different datasets. Here, *Visible* denotes all landmarks within the current imaging field of view and *All* denotes the overall error of all landmarks.

| Dataset | | Results | |
|---------|---------|-----------------|------------------|
| | | $MPJPE_{2D}$ (px) | $MPJPE_{3D}$ (mm) |
| Verse | Visible | 3.17 | 11.62 |
| | All | 4.91 | 14.44 |
| CT | Visible | 5.11 | 27.98 |
| | All | 7.98 | 33.4 |
| CBCT | Visible | 14.85 | 38.01 |

## 4   Discussion and Conclusion

Here, we presented a method for generating a 3D patient specific model of the skeleton using a single X-ray projection image. Our proposed approach from Table 1 delivers a 2-fold improvement in 2D errors compared to the baseline method, and a 16% improvement in 3D errors. The resulting errors when applied to projection images of CBCT (38.01 mm) and CT data (27.98 mm) from Table 2 reveal that our approach, which combines regression and iterative methods, is a reliable starting point for generating bone models from single view X-ray images through statistical models. We note that the errors on CBCT data are greater when compared to those on the CT dataset. This is due to the annotations on the CBCT data being roughly positioned in the image volume, which may not align completely with the actual location corresponding to the BOSS model. We observe that utilizing the iterative optimizer resulted in improved 2D and 3D alignment. Moreover, we found that training the network to optimize the reprojection error was advantageous over solely using iterative optimization during evaluation. Furthermore, we note slightly elevated errors when considering all landmarks as opposed to just the visible landmarks. This is due to the fact that the position of the scapula, clavicle, or any other crucial part cannot be precisely established without the assistance of image information.

In conclusion, we introduced a fast and dependable deep learning-based iterative mesh model generation framework that produces accurate 3D skeletal models from a single X-ray projection image. This framework may allow to generate and precisely locate a digital twin, e.g. generated from the BOSS model, of a patient in an interventional imaging environment, which has great potential in assisting in multiple tasks of image-guided interventions, such as automatic system positioning or automatically adjusting imaging parameters based on body parameters to be imaged. Additionally, it can act as a starting point for 2D/3D image registration methods, after which specialized techniques such as [3] can be utilized. Future work will evaluate these tasks.

**Disclaimer.** The concepts and information presented in this article are based on research and are not commercially available.

# References

1. Ehlke, M., Ramm, H., Lamecker, H., Hege, H.C., Zachow, S.: Fast generation of virtual X-ray images for reconstruction of 3D anatomy. IEEE Trans. Vis. Comput. Graph. **19**(12), 2673–2682 (2013)
2. Fotouhi, J., Liu, X., Armand, M., Navab, N., Unberath, M.: From perspective X-ray imaging to parallax-robust orthographic stitching. arXiv preprint arXiv:2003.02959 (2020)
3. Jaganathan, S., Wang, J., Borsdorf, A., Shetty, K., Maier, A.: Deep iterative 2D/3D registration. In: de Bruijne, M., et al. (eds.) MICCAI 2021. LNCS, vol. 12904, pp. 383–392. Springer, Cham (2021). https://doi.org/10.1007/978-3-030-87202-1_37
4. Kanazawa, A., Black, M.J., Jacobs, D.W., Malik, J.: End-to-end recovery of human shape and pose. In: IEEE Conference on Computer Vision and Pattern Recognition (CVPR), pp. 7122–7131. IEEE Computer Society (2018)
5. Kasten, Y., Doktofsky, D., Kovler, I.: End-to-end convolutional neural network for 3D reconstruction of knee bones from bi-planar X-ray images. In: Deeba, F., Johnson, P., Würfl, T., Ye, J.C. (eds.) MLMIR 2020. LNCS, vol. 12450, pp. 123–133. Springer, Cham (2020). https://doi.org/10.1007/978-3-030-61598-7_12
6. Keller, M., Zuffi, S., Black, M.J., Pujades, S.: OSSO: obtaining skeletal shape from outside. In: Proceedings IEEE/CVF Conference on Computer Vision and Pattern Recognition (CVPR), June 2022, pp. 20492–20501 (2022)

7. Kinahan, P., Muzi, M., Bialecki, B., Herman, B., Coombs, L.: Data from the ACRIN 6668 trial NSCLC-FDG-PET (2019). https://doi.org/10.7937/TCIA.2019.30ILQFCL

8. Kingma, D.P., Ba, J.: Adam: a method for stochastic optimization. arXiv preprint arXiv:1412.6980 (2014)

9. Kolotouros, N., Pavlakos, G., Black, M.J., Daniilidis, K.: Learning to reconstruct 3D human pose and shape via model-fitting in the loop. In: ICCV (2019)

10. Lamecker, H., Wenckebach, T.H., Hege, H.: Atlas-based 3D-shape reconstruction from X-ray images. In: 18th International Conference on Pattern Recognition, ICPR 2006, vol. 1, pp. 371–374 (2006). https://doi.org/10.1109/ICPR.2006.279

11. Li, J., Xu, C., Chen, Z., Bian, S., Yang, L., Lu, C.: HybrIK: a hybrid analytical-neural inverse kinematics solution for 3D human pose and shape estimation. In: Proceedings of the IEEE/CVF Conference on Computer Vision and Pattern Recognition, pp. 3383–3393 (2021)

12. Loper, M., Mahmood, N., Romero, J., Pons-Moll, G., Black, M.J.: SMPL: a skinned multi-person linear model. ACM Trans. Graph. (Proc. SIGGRAPH Asia) **34**(6), 248:1–248:16 (2015)

13. Moon, G., Lee, K.M.: I2L-MeshNet: image-to-lixel prediction network for accurate 3D human pose and mesh estimation from a single RGB image. arXiv arXiv:2008.03713 (2020)

14. Pavlakos, G., et al.: Expressive body capture: 3D hands, face, and body from a single image (2019)

15. Pineda, L., et al.: Theseus: a library for differentiable nonlinear optimization. In: Advances in Neural Information Processing Systems (2022)

16. Roser, P., et al.: Physics-driven learning of x-ray skin dose distribution in interventional procedures. Med. Phys. **46**(10), 4654–4665 (2019)

17. Sekuboyina, A., et al.: VerSe: a vertebrae labelling and segmentation benchmark for multi-detector CT images. Med. Image Anal. **73**, 102166 (2021)

18. Shen, L., Zhao, W., Xing, L.: Patient-specific reconstruction of volumetric computed tomography images from a single projection view via deep learning. Nat. Biomed. Eng. **3**(11), 880–888 (2019)

19. Shetty, K., et al.: BOSS: Bones, organs and skin shape model. Comput. Biol. Med. **165**, 107383 (2023). https://doi.org/10.1016/j.compbiomed.2023.107383. ISSN 0010-4825

20. Shetty, K., et al.: PLIKS: a pseudo-linear inverse kinematic solver for 3D human body estimation. In: Proceedings of the IEEE/CVF Conference on Computer Vision and Pattern Recognition (CVPR), June 2023, pp. 574–584 (2023)

21. Tan, M., Le, Q.: EfficientNetV2: smaller models and faster training. In: International Conference on Machine Learning, pp. 10096–10106. PMLR (2021)

22. Tretschk, E., et al.: State of the art in dense monocular non-rigid 3D reconstruction (2022). https://doi.org/10.48550/ARXIV.2210.15664. https://arxiv.org/abs/2210.15664

23. Unberath, M., et al.: DeepDRR – a catalyst for machine learning in fluoroscopy-guided procedures. In: Frangi, A.F., Schnabel, J.A., Davatzikos, C., Alberola-López, C., Fichtinger, G. (eds.) MICCAI 2018. LNCS, vol. 11073, pp. 98–106. Springer, Cham (2018). https://doi.org/10.1007/978-3-030-00937-3_12

24. Vávra, P., et al.: Recent development of augmented reality in surgery: a review. J. Healthc. Eng. **2017**, 4574172 (2017)

25. Ying, X., Guo, H., Ma, K., Wu, J., Weng, Z., Zheng, Y.: X2CT-GAN: reconstructing CT from biplanar X-rays with generative adversarial networks (2019)

26. Zheng, C., et al.: Deep learning-based human pose estimation: a survey. arXiv arXiv:2012.13392 (2020)

# GastroVision: A Multi-class Endoscopy Image Dataset for Computer Aided Gastrointestinal Disease Detection

Debesh Jha[1]([✉]), Vanshali Sharma[2], Neethi Dasu[3], Nikhil Kumar Tomar[1], Steven Hicks[4], M. K. Bhuyan[2], Pradip K. Das[2], Michael A. Riegler[4], Pål Halvorsen[4], Ulas Bagci[1], and Thomas de Lange[5,6]

[1] Department of Radiology, Northwestern University, Chicago, USA
{debesh.jha,nikhil.tomar,ulas.bagci}@northwestern.edu
[2] Indian Institute of Technology Guwahati, Assam, India
{vanshalisharma,mkb,pkdas}@iitg.ac.in
[3] Department of Gastroenterology, Jefferson Health, Cherry Hill, NJ, USA
[4] SimulaMet, Oslo, Norway
{steven,michael,paalh}@simula.no
[5] Department of Medicine and Emergencies - Mölndal Sahlgrenska University Hospital, Region Västra Götaland, Mölndal, Sweden
thomas.de.lange@gu.se
[6] Department of Molecular and Clinical Medicine, Sahlgrenska Academy, University of Gothenburg, Gothenburg, Sweden

**Abstract.** Integrating real-time artificial intelligence (AI) systems in clinical practices faces challenges such as scalability and acceptance. These challenges include data availability, biased outcomes, data quality, lack of transparency, and underperformance on unseen datasets from different distributions. The scarcity of large-scale, precisely labeled, and diverse datasets are the major challenge for clinical integration. This scarcity is also due to the legal restrictions and extensive manual efforts required for accurate annotations from clinicians. To address these challenges, we present *GastroVision*, a multi-center open-access gastrointestinal (GI) endoscopy dataset that includes different anatomical landmarks, pathological abnormalities, polyp removal cases and normal findings (a total of 27 classes) from the GI tract. The dataset comprises 8,000 images acquired from Bærum Hospital in Norway and Karolinska University Hospital in Sweden and was annotated and verified by experienced GI endoscopists. Furthermore, we validate the significance of our dataset with extensive benchmarking based on the popular deep learning based baseline models. We believe our dataset can facilitate the development of AI-based algorithms for GI disease detection and classification. Our dataset is available at https://osf.io/84e7f/.

**Keywords:** Medical image · GastroVision · Gastrointestinal diseases

D. Jha and V. Sharma—These authors contributed equally to this work.
U. Bagci and T. de Lange—Shared senior authorship.

A. K. Maier et al. (Eds.): ML4MHD 2023, LNCS 14315, pp. 125–140, 2024.
https://doi.org/10.1007/978-3-031-47679-2_10

# 1    Introduction

Gastrointestinal (GI) cancers account for 26% of cancer incidences and 35% of cancer-related deaths worldwide. In 2018, there were approximately 4.8 million new cases of GI cancer and 3.4 million deaths [7]. The five major types of GI cancers are colo-rectal (1.93 million cases; third most common cancer), pancreas (466,003 deaths; lowest survival rate), liver (905,677 cases), stomach (1.09 million cases), and esophagus (604,100 cases) [13]. These cancer cases are predicted to increase by 58%, and related deaths could show a 73% rise by 2040 [7]. Early detection of such cancers and their precursors can play an important role in improving the outcome and make the treatment less invasive. Some of the common examinations performed for GI cancer detection include endoscopy or esophagogastroduodenoscopy (EGD), capsule endoscopy, colonoscopy, imaging studies (MRI, X-ray, ultrasound, CT scan, or PET scan) or endoscopic ultrasound (EUS). Endoscopy is widely accepted as the gold standard for detecting abnormalities of the bowel lumen and mucosa, upper endoscopy for esophagus, stomach, and the duodenum and colonoscopy for the large bowel and rectum GI tract for abnormalities, respectively.

The endoscopies are performed by nurses or doctor endoscopists. The assessment of the endoscopy examinations is operator dependent, and the assessment and therapeutic decision vary between endoscopists. Consequently, the quality and accuracy of detection and diagnosis of lesions are attributed to the level of the operator skills and efforts of the endoscopists. Despite various measures taken to provide guidance for operators, significant lesion miss rates are still reported. For example, there is evidence of colon polyp miss rates of up to 27% due to polyps and operator characteristics [2,20]. Considering the shortcomings of the manual review process, various automated systems are adopted to provide AI-based real-time support to clinicians to reduce lesion miss rates and misinterpretation of lesions to ultimately increase detection rates. A microsimulation study reports a 4.8% incremental gain in the reduction of colorectal cancer incidence when colonoscopy screening was combined with AI tools [6]. Such findings motivated research work in healthcare to adopt AI as a potential tool for GI cancer detection. Gastric cancer, inflammatory bowel disease (IBD), and esophageal neoplasia are some of the GI tract findings already being investigated using AI techniques [1]. Despite AI being adopted in some hospitals for clinical applications, the integration of AI into the extensive clinical setting is still limited. Integrating AI techniques with regular clinical practices is multifactorial and poses serious concerns regarding its implementation in large-scale healthcare systems. One of the significant factors is the algorithmic bias, which worsens when the system learns from the annotations handled by a single, non-blinded endoscopist who may have personal thresholds to label the findings.

Moreover, most existing AI models depend on data acquired from a single center, which makes them less valid when faced with a varied patient population. This leads to spectrum bias under which AI systems encounter performance drops due to the significant shift in the original clinical context and the test sample population. In such cases, unexpected outcomes and diagnostic accuracy could be obtained using automated tools. Such bias issues could reach the clinical systems at any point of the process, including data collection, study design, data entry and pre-processing, algorithm design, and implementation. The very beginning of the process, i.e., data collection, is of utmost importance for reproducibility and to perform validations on images from a diverse population, different centers, and imaging modalities. To develop scalable healthcare systems, it is vital to consider these challenges and perform real-time validations. However, the scarcity of comprehensive data covering a range of real-time imaging scenarios arising during endoscopy or colonoscopy makes it difficult to develop a robust AI-based model. Although much progress has been made on automated cancer detection and classification [16,19], it is still challenging to adapt such models into real-time clinical settings as they are tested on small-sized datasets with limited classes.

Some classes in the dataset could be scarce because some conditions or diseases occur less often. Consequently, such findings are not frequently captured and remain unexplored despite requiring medical attention. AI-based detection of these findings, even with a small sample count, can significantly benefit from techniques like one-shot or few-shot learning. These techniques allow the AI models to learn patterns and features indicative of the condition, thus, enabling accurate diagnosis with minimal training data. Apart from the above-mentioned limitations, many existing datasets are available on request, and prior consenting is required, which delays the process and does not guarantee accessibility. Therefore, in this paper, we publish *GastroVision*, an open-access multi-class endoscopy image dataset for automated GI disease detection that does not require prior consenting and can be downloaded easily with a single click. The data covers a wide range of classes that can allow initial exploration of many anatomical landmarks and pathological findings.

The main contributions of this work are summarized below:

- We present an open-access multi-class GI endoscopy dataset, namely, *Gastrovision*, containing 8,000 images with 27 classes from two hospitals in Norway and Sweden. The dataset exhibits a diverse range of classes, including anatomical landmarks, pathological findings, polyp removal cases and normal or regular findings. It covers a wide range of clinical scenarios encountered in endoscopic procedures.
- We evaluated a series of deep learning baseline models on standard evaluation metrics using our proposed dataset. With this baseline, we invite the research community to improve our results and develop novel GI endoscopy solutions on our comprehensive set of GI finding classes. Additionally, we encourage computer vision and machine learning researchers to validate their methods on our open-access data for a fair comparison. This can aid in developing state-of-the-art solutions and computer-aided systems for GI disease detection and other general machine learning classification tasks.

**Table 1.** List of the existing datasets within GI endoscopy.

| Dataset | Data type | Size | Accessibility |
|---|---|---|---|
| Kvasir-SEG [17] | Polyps | 1,000 images[†][♣] | Public |
| HyperKvasir [11] | GI findings | 110,079 images & 374 videos | Public |
| Kvasir-Capsule [24] | GI findings[◇] | 4,741,504 images | Public |
| Kvasir [22] | GI findings | 8,000 images | Public |
| CVC-ColonDB [10] | Polyps | 380 images[†] [‡] | As per request[•] |
| ETIS-Larib Polyp DB [23] | Polyps | 196 images[†] | Public |
| EDD2020 [3,4] | GI lesions | 386 images[†][♣] | Public |
| CVC-ClinicDB [9] | Polyps | 612 images[†] | Public |
| CVC-VideoClinicDB [8] | Polyps | 11,954 images[†] | As per request |
| ASU-Mayo polyp database [25] | Polyps | 18,781 images[†] | As per request[•] |
| KID [18] | Angiectasia, bleeding, inflammations[◇] | > 2500 images, 47 videos | Public[•] |
| PolypGen [5] | Polyps | 1,537 images[†][♣] & 2,225 video sequence, 4,275 negative frame | Public |
| SUN Database [21] | Polyps | 158,690 video frames[♣] | As per request |
| **GastroVision (ours)** | GI findings | 8,000 image frames | Public |

[†]Segmentation ground truth    [•]Not available now  [‡]Contour    [◇]Video capsule endoscopy    [♣] Bounding box information

## 2  Related Work

Table 1 shows the list of the existing dataset along with data type, their size, and accessibility. It can be observed that most of the existing datasets in the literature are from colonoscopy procedures and consist of polyps still frames or videos. These are mostly used for segmentation tasks. Most of the existing datasets are small in size and do not capture some critical anatomical landmarks or pathological findings. In the earlier GI detection works, the CVC-ClinicDB [9] and CVC-ColonDB [10] were widely used. **CVC-ClinicDB** is developed from 23 colonoscopy video studies acquired with white light. These videos provide 31 video sequences, each containing one polyp, which finally generates 612 images of size 576 × 768. **CVC-ColonDB** consists of 300 different images obtained from 15 random cases. Similarly, **ETIS-Larib Polyp DB** [23] is a colonoscopy dataset consisting of 196 polyp frames and their corresponding segmentation masks. Recently, **Kvasir-SEG** [17] dataset has been introduced that comprises of 1,000 colonoscopy images with segmentation ground truth and bounding box coordinate details. This dataset offers a diverse range of polyp frames, including multiple diminutive polyps, small-sized polyps, regular polyps, sessile or flat polyps collected from varied cohort populations. The dataset is open-access and is one of the most commonly used datasets for automatic polyp segmentation.

The **ASU-Mayo Clinic Colonoscopy Video (c) database** [25] is a copyrighted dataset and is considered the first largest collection of short and long video sequences. Its training set is composed of 10 positive shots with polyps inside and 10 negative shots with no polyps. The associated test set is provided with 18 different unannotated videos. **CVC-VideoClinicDB** [8] is extracted from more than 40 long and short video sequences. Its training set comprises 18 different sequences with an approximate segmentation ground truth and Paris classification for each polyp. **SUN Colonoscopy Video Database** comprises 49,136 polyp frames and 109,554 non-polyp frames. Unlike the datasets described above, this dataset includes pathological classification labels, polyp size, and shape information. It also includes bounding box coordinate details. The **Polyp-**

Gen [5] dataset is an open-access dataset that comprises 1,537 polyp images, 2,225 positive video sequences, and 4,275 negative frames. The dataset is collected from six different centers in Europe and Africa. Altogether the dataset provides 3,762 positive frames and 4,275 negative frames. These still images and video frames are collected from varied populations, endoscopic systems, and surveillance expert in Norway, France, United Kingdom, Egypt, and Italy and is one of the comprehensive open-access datasets for polyp detection and segmentation.

Apart from the lower GI-related datasets, there are a few datasets that provide combined samples of upper and lower GI findings. For example, **HyperKvasir** [11] is a multi-class GI endoscopy dataset that covers 23 classes of anatomical landmarks. It contains 110,079 images out of which 10,662 are labeled and 99,417 are unlabeled images. The **EDD2020** dataset [3,4] is a collection of five classes and 386 still images with detection and segmentation ground truth. The classes are divided into 160 non-dysplastic Barrett's, 88 suspicious precancerous lesions, 74 high-grade dysplasia, 53 cancer, and 127 polyps with overall 503 ground truth annotations. The **Kvasir-Capsule** [24] is a video capsule endoscopy dataset comprising 4,741,504 image frames extracted from 117 videos. From the total frames, 4,694,266 are unlabeled, and 47,238 frames are annotated with a bounding box for each of the 14 classes. Similarly, **KID** [18] is a capsule endoscopy dataset with 47 videos and over 2,500 images. The images are annotated for normal, vascular, inflammatory, lymphangiectasias, and polypoid lesions.

The literature review shows that most GI-related datasets focus on a single specific finding, such as colon polyps. Some of the datasets are small in size and have ignored non-lesion frames, which are essential for developing algorithms to be integrated into clinical settings. Additionally, many of these datasets are available on request and require approval from the data providers resulting in further delays. A few datasets like Kvasir, HyperKvasir, Kvasir-Capsule and KID provide multiple GI findings. However, Kvasir-Capsule and KID are video capsule endoscopy datasets. The Kvasir dataset has only eight classes, whereas Hyperkvasir has 23 classes. In contrast, our *GastroVision* dataset has 27 classes and covers more labeled classes of anatomical landmarks, pathological findings, and normal findings. Additionally, we establish baseline results on this dataset for GI disease detection and classification, offering valuable research resources for advancing GI endoscopy studies.

## 3    GastroVision

Here, we provide detailed information about the dataset, acquisition protocol, ethical and privacy aspects of data and suggested metrics.

### 3.1    Dataset Details

GastroVision is an open-access dataset that incorporates 8,000 images pertaining to 27 different labeled classes (Fig. 1). Most images are obtained through

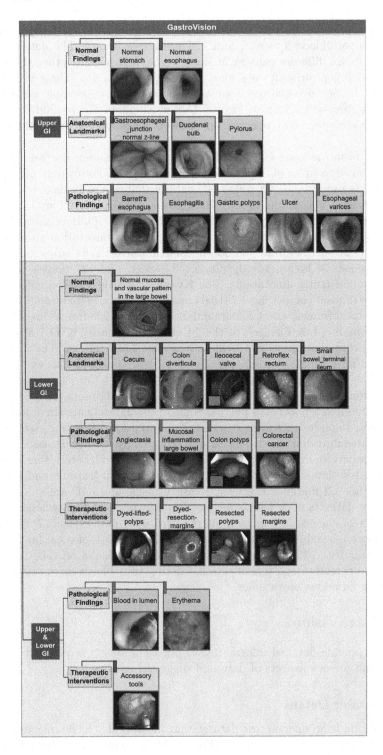

**Fig. 1.** Example images from the gastrointestinal tract showing distinct findings from the upper and lower GI tract.

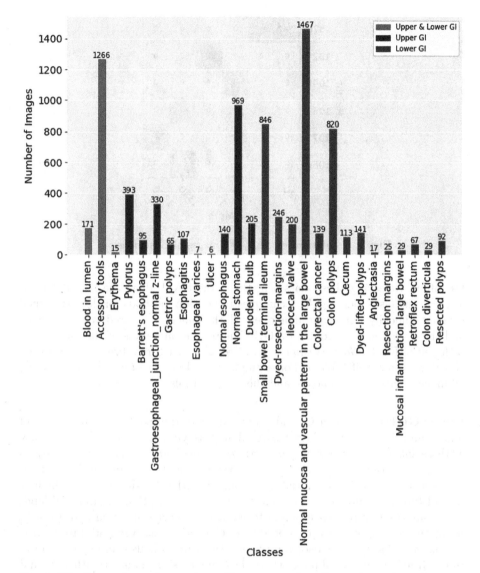

**Fig. 2.** The figure shows the number of images per class. Some classes have few samples because of the rarity of the findings and the technical challenges associated with obtaining such samples in endoscopic settings.

White Light Imaging (WLI), while a few samples are acquired using Narrow Band Imaging (NBI). These classes are categorized into two broad categories: *Upper GI tract* and *Lower GI tract*. The number of images under each class is presented in Fig. 2. These classes indicate findings acquired from GI tract. It can be observed that the sample count is not balanced across classes, which is generally experienced in the medical image acquisition process as some findings occur

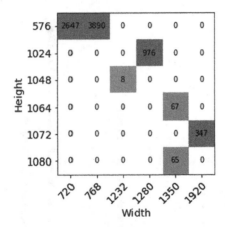

**Fig. 3.** Resolutions of the 8,000 images of GastroVision.

less often. Releasing these classes in the dataset will allow the researchers to leverage the fast-emerging AI techniques to develop methods for detecting such rare but clinically significant anomalies. All the images are stored in JPG format, and the overall size is around 1.8 GB. The resolution details of the images can be found in Fig. 3. *GastroVision* is provided as a structured directory, with each class having a specific folder. For example, the '*Accessory tools*' folder contains all images featuring diagnostic and therapeutic tools.

**Upper GI Tract:** Upper GI endoscopy examines the esophagus, stomach, and duodenum. The various classes covered in this GI tract are discussed below as three subcategories: *normal findings, anatomical landmarks*, and *pathological findings*. A detailed categorization is shown in Fig. 1. The **normal stomach** serves as a critical site for initial digestion, while the **duodenal bulb**, the first part of the small intestine, is critical for nutrient absorption. Anatomical landmarks are used as reference points to indicate a specific location and assist in navigating during endoscopy procedures. The **gastroesophageal junction** is an anatomical area where **esophagus** joins the **stomach** also alining to the **normal z-line**, a transitional point where the esophagus's squamous epithelium and the stomach's columnar mucosa lining join. **Pylorus** is a sphincter connecting the stomach and the duodenum, the first part of the small intestine.

Apart from these anatomical landmarks, any pathological conditions may be encountered during endoscopy. **Esophagitis**, the most common abnormality, is characterized by an inflammation of the esophagus. This disease is graded based on its severity according to the Los Angeles classification. For example, grade B refers to the condition when the mucosal break is limited to the mucosal fold and is more than 5 mm long. In grade D, mucosal break affects 75% of the esophageal circumference. Long standing esophagitis may cause **Barett's esophagus**, a condition in which the cells of the esophagus's lining start to change, and tissues appear red. This is a precancerous condition. Other frequent lesions observed are **polyps**, abnormal tissue growth or ulcers. **Gastric polyps** are abnormal growths in the stomach lining. **Ulcers** are the open sores in the stomach or duodenum that can lead to discomfort and bleeding. **Esophageal varices** result from portal hypertension, causing swollen veins in the esophagus. **Erythema** refers to redness, often indicating inflammation and **blood in the lumen** denotes bleeding. **Accessory tools** aid in investigating and diagnosing upper and lower GI tract conditions for targeted treatment.

**Lower GI Tract:** The lower GI tract is examined by colonoscopy to investigate any abnormalities in the colon, the rectum, and the terminal ileum (the last part of the small bowel). Here, we covered one more subcategory, *therapeutic interventions*, in addition to *normal findings*, *anatomical landmarks*, and *pathological findings*. A detailed class-wise division is shown in Fig. 1.

The **normal mucosa and vascular pattern in the large bowel** is essential for absorbing water and electrolytes. The different anatomical landmarks associated with lower GI include **cecum** (first part of the large intestine), visualizing the appendiceal orifice, **ileocecal valve** (sphincter muscle between ileum and colon), and the **small bowel**. During the colonoscopy, these anatomical landmarks act as reference points to prove complete examination. Retroflexion in the rectum is performed to visualize a blind zone, using the bending section of the colonoscope to visualize the distal area of the colon, called **rectroflex-rectum**. The **terminal ileum**, the last part of the small intestine, aids in nutrient absorption. **Colon diverticula**, small pouch-like protrusions, can form along the colon's weakened wall, often in the sigmoid colon [12].

During the colonoscopy, the endoscopist navigates through these landmarks and looks for abnormalities such as **polyps**, **angiectasia**, and inflammation like **ulcerative colitis**. **Angiectasia** is a common lesion representing abnormal blood vessels and is responsible for obscure recurrent lower GI bleeding. These can easily be distinguished from the **normal vessels** shown in Fig. 1. **Colorectal cancer** occurs in the colon or rectum. One of the early signs of this colorectal cancer can be detected through **colon polyps**. **Mucosal inflammation in the large bowel** may be caused by different factors, such as infections or chronic inflammatory conditions.

Apart from the aforementioned pathological conditions, several therapeutic interventions are adopted to treat the detected anomalies effectively. It frequently involves the removal of the lesion/polyp. The surrounding of such **resected polyps**, also called the **resection margins** or resection sites, are then considered for biopsies. To enhance lesion demarcation, a solution containing indigo carmine is injected, making resection easier. The appearance of blue color underneath the **dyed-lifted-polyp** provides accurate polyp margins. After resecting such polyps, the underlying region, known as **dyed-resection-margin**, appears blue. These margins are important to examine for any remaining tissue of the resected polyp.

## 3.2    Dataset Acquisition, Collection and Construction

**Data Acquisition and Collection:** The dataset images are acquired from two centers (Department of Gastroenterology, Bærum Hospital, Vestre Viken Hospital Trust (VV), Norway and Karolinska University Hospital, Stockholm, Sweden) using standard endoscopy equipment from Olympus (Olympus Europe, Germany) and Pentax (Pentax Medical Europe, Germany). A team of expert gastroenterologists, one junior doctor, and two computational scientists were involved in the labelling of the images and the related review process. It is worth noting that for dataset collection, we labeled some of the unlabeled images from the HyperKvasir dataset and included them in our dataset. Additionally, we labeled the images acquired from the Karolinska University Hospital to their respective classes for developing a diverse and multi-center "GastroVision" dataset.

**Ethical and Privacy Aspects of the Data:** The dataset is constructed while preserving the patients' anonymity and privacy. All videos and images from Bærum hospitals were fully anonymized, following the GDPR requirements for full anonymization. Hence, it is exempted from patient consent. The files were renamed using randomly generated filenames. The Norwegian Privacy Data Protection Authority approved this export of anonymized images for research purposes. As the dataset development procedure involved no interference with the medical treatment or care of the patient, it has also been granted an exemption for approval by Regional Committee for Medical and Health Research Ethics - South East Norway. Similarly, the data collection process at Karolinska University Hospital, Sweden, is completely anonymized as per the GDPR requirements.

## 3.3    Suggested Metrics

Standard multi-class classification metrics, such as Matthews Correlation Coefficient (MCC), micro and macro averages of recall/sensitivity, precision, and F1-score, can be used to validate the performance using our dataset. MCC provides a balanced measure even in cases with largely varying class sizes. A macro-average will compute the metric independently for each class and then take the average, whereas a micro-average will aggregate the contributions of all classes to compute the metric. Recall presents the ratio of correctly predicted positive observations to all the original observations in the actual class. Precision is the ratio of correctly predicted positive observations to all the positive predicted observations. F1-score integrates both recall and precision and calculates a weighted average/harmonic mean of these two metrics.

**Table 2.** Results for all classification experiments on the Gastrovision dataset.

| Method | Macro Average | | | Micro Average | | | MCC |
|---|---|---|---|---|---|---|---|
| | Prec. | Recall | F1 | Prec. | Recall | F1 | |
| ResNet-50 [14] | 0.4373 | 0.4379 | 0.4330 | 0.6816 | 0.6816 | 0.6816 | 0.6416 |
| Pre-trained ResNet-152 [14] | 0.5258 | 0.4287 | 0.4496 | 0.6879 | 0.6879 | 0.6879 | 0.6478 |
| Pre-trained EfficientNet-B0 [26] | 0.5285 | 0.4326 | 0.4519 | 0.6759 | 0.6759 | 0.6759 | 0.6351 |
| Pre-trained DenseNet-169 [15] | 0.6075 | 0.4603 | 0.4883 | 0.7055 | 0.7055 | 0.7055 | 0.6685 |
| Pre-trained ResNet-50 [14] | 0.6398 | 0.6073 | 0.6176 | 0.8146 | 0.8146 | 0.8146 | 0.7921 |
| Pre-trained DenseNet-121 [15] | **0.7388** | **0.6231** | **0.6504** | **0.8203** | **0.8203** | **0.8203** | **0.7987** |

# 4  Experiments and Results

In this section, we describe the implementation details, technical validation and the limitation of the dataset.

## 4.1  Implementation Details

All deep learning diagnostic models are trained on NVIDIA TITAN Xp GPU using PyTorch 1.12.1 framework. A stratified sampling is performed to preserve the similar distribution of each class during 60:20:20 training, validation, and testing split formation. The images are resized to 224 × 224 pixels, and simple data augmentations, including random rotation and random horizontal flip, are applied. All models are configured with similar hyperparameters, and a learning rate of $1e^{-4}$ is initially set with 150 epochs. An Adam optimizer is used with the *ReduceLROnPlateau* scheduler. More description about the implementation details and dataset can be found on our GitHub page[1].

## 4.2  Technical Validation

To evaluate the presented data for technical quality and classification tasks, we performed a series of experiments using some state-of-the-art deep learning models. The purpose of this preliminary validation is to provide baseline results that can be referred to for comparison by future researchers. We carried out multi-class classification using CNN-based models, namely, ResNet-50 [14], ResNet-152 [14], EfficientNet-B0 [26], DenseNet-121 [15], and DenseNet-169 [15], considering their competent performance in GI-related image-based tasks in the literature [27]. Note that we have only included classes with more than 25 samples in the experiments, which resulted in 22 classes in total. However, we also release the other classes with fewer samples to welcome new interesting findings in areas similar to one-shot learning.

---

[1] https://github.com/DebeshJha/GastroVision.

**Table 3.** Class-wise performance associated with the best outcome obtained using pre-trained DenseNet-121.

| Class | Pre-trained DenseNet-121 | | | Support |
|---|---|---|---|---|
| | Precision | Recall | F1-score | |
| Accessory tools | 0.93 | 0.96 | 0.95 | 253 |
| Barrett's esophagus | 0.55 | 0.32 | 0.4 | 19 |
| Blood in lumen | 0.86 | 0.91 | 0.89 | 34 |
| Cecum | 0.33 | 0.17 | 0.23 | 23 |
| Colon diverticula | 1 | 0.33 | 0.5 | 6 |
| Colon polyps | 0.78 | 0.87 | 0.82 | 163 |
| Colorectal cancer | 0.63 | 0.41 | 0.5 | 29 |
| Duodenal bulb | 0.72 | 0.76 | 0.74 | 41 |
| Dyed-lifted-polyps | 0.86 | 0.86 | 0.86 | 28 |
| Dyed-resection-margins | 0.94 | 0.92 | 0.93 | 49 |
| Esophagitis | 0.5 | 0.23 | 0.31 | 22 |
| Gastric polyps | 0.6 | 0.23 | 0.33 | 13 |
| Gastroesophageal_junction_normal z-line | 0.65 | 0.85 | 0.74 | 66 |
| Ileocecal valve | 0.74 | 0.7 | 0.72 | 40 |
| Mucosal inflammation large bowel | 1 | 0.33 | 0.5 | 6 |
| Normal esophagus | 0.72 | 0.82 | 0.77 | 28 |
| Normal mucosa and vasular pattern in the large bowel | 0.81 | 0.87 | 0.84 | 293 |
| Normal stomach | 0.9 | 0.86 | 0.88 | 194 |
| Pylorus | 0.8 | 0.92 | 0.86 | 78 |
| Resected polyps | 0.33 | 0.11 | 0.17 | 18 |
| Retroflex rectum | 0.75 | 0.43 | 0.55 | 14 |
| Small bowel_terminal ileum | 0.86 | 0.85 | 0.85 | 169 |

The different experiments performed include *(a) ResNet-50*: The model is randomly initialized, and an end-to-end training is done, *(b) Pre-trained ResNet-50* and *(c) Pre-trained DenseNet-121*: The models are initialized with pre-trained weights, and then all layers are fine-tuned, *(d) Pre-trained ResNet-152*, *(e) Pre-trained EfficientNet-B0* and *(f) Pre-trained DenseNet-169*: The models are initialized with pre-trained weights, and only the updated last layer is fine-tuned. All the above pre-trained models use ImageNet weights. The associated results are shown in Table 2. It can be observed that the best outcome is obtained using the pre-trained DenseNet-121. A class-wise analysis using the same model is provided in Table 3 and Fig. 4. It shows that while most classes achieved satisfactory prediction outcomes, a few proved to be very challenging for the classification model. For a more detailed analysis, we plotted a two-dimensional t-SNE embedding for *GastroVision* (Fig. 5). The classes like *Normal stomach, Dyed-resection-margins*, which present a clear distinction in the t-SNE embedding, are less often misclassified. The above points could be the

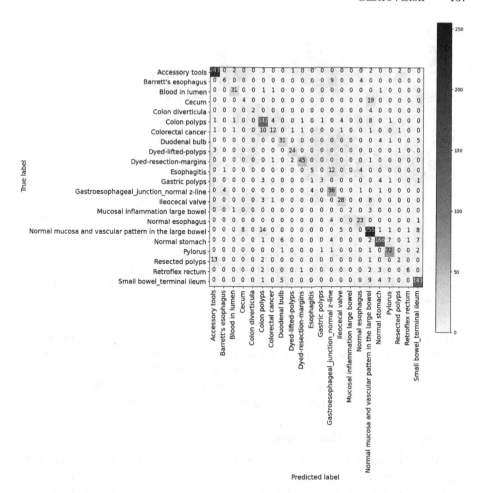

**Fig. 4.** Confusion matrix for the best outcome obtained using pre-trained DenseNet-121.

reasons for the F1-score of 0.88 and 0.93 in the case of *Dyed-resection-margins* and *Normal stomach* classes, respectively. On the other hand, there are some overlapping classes such as *Cecum* and *Normal mucosa and vascular pattern in the large bowel* or *Colorectal cancer* and *Colon polyps* which do not present clear demarcation with each other and hence, are likely to be misclassified.

Considering the overall results and many overlapping classes (without distinct clustering), it can be inferred that classifying GI-related anatomical landmarks and pathological findings is very challenging. Many abnormalities are hard to differentiate, and the rarely occurring findings have higher chances of getting misclassified. This presents the challenge of developing a robust AI system that could address multiple aspects important for GI image classification, e.g., many findings are subtle and difficult to be identified, and some findings are not easily

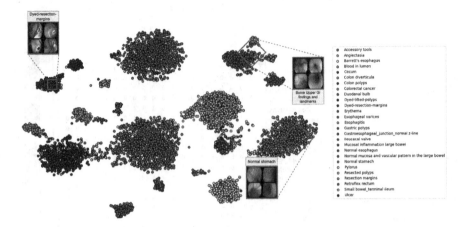

**Fig. 5.** Two-dimensional t-SNE embedding for GastroVision. The pre-trained DenseNet-121 model, which is further trained on our training set, is used to extract features. Some sample images are shown with either a specific or a broader (due to multiple overlapping classes) categorization.

acquired during the endoscopy procedure, which results in less number of data samples. Such underrepresented classes need to be explored with some specific algorithms specially designed to leverage the availability of a few hard-to-find samples. Thus, the potential of the baseline results and associated issues and challenges motivate the need to publish this dataset for further investigations.

### 4.3   Limitation of the Dataset

Our dataset, *GastroVision*, is a unique and diverse dataset with the potential to explore a wide range of anatomical and pathological findings using automated diagnosis. Although this labeled image data can enable the researchers to develop methods to detect GI-related abnormalities and other landmarks, it lacks segmented annotations in the current version, which could further enhance the treatment experience and surgical procedures. It is important to note that some classes (for example, colon diverticula, erythema, cecum, esophagitis, esophageal varices, ulcer and pylorus) have only a few images. Despite this limitation, our dataset is well suited for one-shot and few-shot learning approaches to explore some GI-related conditions that have still not received attention in medical image analysis. In the future, we plan to extend the dataset by including more classes and a larger number of samples, along with ground truth for some of the classes that could be used for segmentation purposes as well as images with higher resolution from the most recent endoscopy systems.

## 5   Conclusion

In this paper, we presented a new multi-class endoscopy dataset, *GastroVision*, for GI anomalies and disease detection. We have made the dataset available for the research community along with the implementation details of our method. The labeled image data can allow researchers to formulate methodologies for classifying different GI findings, such as important pathological lesions, endoscopic polyp removal cases, and anatomical landmarks found in the GI tract. We evaluated the dataset using some baseline models and standard multi-class classification metrics. The results motivate the need to investigate better specific techniques for GI-related data. Having a diverse set of categories labeled by expert endoscopists from two different centers, *GastroVision* is unique and valuable for computer-aided GI anomaly and disease detection, patient examinations, and medical training.

**Acknowledgements.** D. Jha is supported by the NIH funding: R01-CA246704 and R01-CA240639. V. Sharma is supported by the INSPIRE fellowship (IF190362), DST, Govt. of India.

# References

1. Abadir, A.P., Ali, M.F., Karnes, W., Samarasena, J.B.: Artificial intelligence in gastrointestinal endoscopy. Clin. Endosc. **53**(2), 132–141 (2020)
2. Ahn, S.B., Han, D.S., Bae, J.H., Byun, T.J., Kim, J.P., Eun, C.S.: The miss rate for colorectal adenoma determined by quality-adjusted, back-to-back colonoscopies. Gut Liver **6**(1), 64 (2012)
3. Ali, S., et al.: Deep learning for detection and segmentation of artefact and disease instances in gastrointestinal endoscopy. Med. Image Anal. **70**, 102002 (2021)
4. Ali, S., et al.: Endoscopy disease detection challenge 2020. arXiv preprint arXiv:2003.03376 (2020)
5. Ali, S., et al.: A multi-centre polyp detection and segmentation dataset for generalisability assessment. Sci. Data **10**(1), 75 (2023)
6. Areia, M., et al.: Cost-effectiveness of artificial intelligence for screening colonoscopy: a modelling study. Lancet Digit. Health **4**(6), e436–e444 (2022)
7. Arnold, M., et al.: Global burden of 5 major types of gastrointestinal cancer. Gastroenterology **159**(1), 335–349 (2020)
8. Bernal, J., Aymeric, H.: MICCAI endoscopic vision challenge polyp detection and segmentation (2017)
9. Bernal, J., Sánchez, F.J., Fernández-Esparrach, G., Gil, D., Rodríguez, C., Vilariño, F.: WM-DOVA maps for accurate polyp highlighting in colonoscopy: validation vs. saliency maps from physicians. Comput. Med. Imaging Graph. **43**, 99–111 (2015)
10. Bernal, J., Sánchez, J., Vilarino, F.: Towards automatic polyp detection with a polyp appearance model. Pattern Recogn. **45**(9), 3166–3182 (2012)
11. Borgli, H., et al.: Hyperkvasir, a comprehensive multi-class image and video dataset for gastrointestinal endoscopy. Sci. Data **7**(1), 1–14 (2020)
12. Crafa, P., Diaz-Cano, S.J.: Changes in colonic structure and mucosal inflammation. In: Colonic Diverticular Disease, pp. 41–61 (2022)
13. Globocan: Cancer today (2020). https://gco.iarc.fr/today/fact-sheets-cancers
14. He, K., Zhang, X., Ren, S., Sun, J.: Deep residual learning for image recognition. In: Proceedings of the IEEE Conference on Computer Vision and Pattern Recognition (CVPR), pp. 770–778 (2016)

15. Huang, G., Liu, Z., Van Der Maaten, L., Weinberger, K.Q.: Densely connected convolutional networks. In: Proceedings of the IEEE Conference on Computer Vision and Pattern Recognition, pp. 4700–4708 (2017)
16. Jha, D., et al.: Real-time polyp detection, localization and segmentation in colonoscopy using deep learning. IEEE Access **9**, 40496–40510 (2021)
17. Jha, D., et al.: Kvasir-SEG: a segmented polyp dataset. In: Proceedings of the International Conference on Multimedia Modeling (MMM), pp. 451–462 (2020)
18. Koulaouzidis, A., et al.: Kid project: an internet-based digital video atlas of capsule endoscopy for research purposes. Endosc. Int. Open **5**(6), E477 (2017)
19. Li, K., et al.: Colonoscopy polyp detection and classification: dataset creation and comparative evaluations. arXiv preprint arXiv:2104.10824 (2021)
20. Mahmud, N., Cohen, J., Tsourides, K., Berzin, T.M.: Computer vision and augmented reality in gastrointestinal endoscopy. Gastroenterol. Rep. **3**(3), 179–184 (2015)
21. Misawa, M., et al.: Development of a computer-aided detection system for colonoscopy and a publicly accessible large colonoscopy video database (with video). Gastrointest. Endosc. **93**(4), 960–967 (2021)
22. Pogorelov, K., et al.: Kvasir: a multi-class image dataset for computer aided gastrointestinal disease detection. In: Proceedings of the 8th ACM on Multimedia Systems Conference, pp. 164–169 (2017)
23. Silva, J., Histace, A., Romain, O., Dray, X., Granado, B.: Toward embedded detection of polyps in WCE images for early diagnosis of colorectal cancer. Int. J. Comput. Assist. Radiol. Surg. **9**(2), 283–293 (2014)
24. Smedsrud, P.H., et al.: Kvasir-capsule, a video capsule endoscopy dataset. Sci. Data **8**(1), 1–10 (2021)
25. Tajbakhsh, N., Gurudu, S.R., Liang, J.: Automated polyp detection in colonoscopy videos using shape and context information. IEEE Trans. Med. Imaging **35**(2), 630–644 (2015)
26. Tan, M., Le, Q.: Efficientnet: rethinking model scaling for convolutional neural networks. In: Proceedings of the International Conference on Machine Learning, pp. 6105–6114 (2019)
27. Thambawita, V., et al.: The medico-task 2018: disease detection in the gastrointestinal tract using global features and deep learning. In: Proceedings of the MediaEval 2018 Workshop (2018)

# MaxCorrMGNN: A Multi-graph Neural Network Framework for Generalized Multimodal Fusion of Medical Data for Outcome Prediction

Niharika S. D'Souza[1]([✉]), Hongzhi Wang[1], Andrea Giovannini[2],
Antonio Foncubierta-Rodriguez[2], Kristen L. Beck[1], Orest Boyko[3],
and Tanveer Syeda-Mahmood[1]

[1] IBM Research Almaden, San Jose, CA, USA
Niharika.Dsouza@ibm.com
[2] IBM Research, Zurich, Switzerland
[3] Department of Radiology, VA Southern Nevada Healthcare System, Las Vegas, NV, USA

**Abstract.** With the emergence of multimodal electronic health records, the evidence for an outcome may be captured across multiple modalities ranging from clinical to imaging and genomic data. Predicting outcomes effectively requires fusion frameworks capable of modeling fine-grained and multi-faceted complex interactions between modality features within and across patients. We develop an innovative fusion approach called MaxCorr MGNN that models non-linear modality correlations within and across patients through Hirschfeld-Gebelein-Reñyi maximal correlation (MaxCorr) embeddings, resulting in a multi-layered graph that preserves the identities of the modalities and patients. We then design, for the first time, a generalized multi-layered graph neural network (MGNN) for task-informed reasoning in multi-layered graphs, that learns the parameters defining patient-modality graph connectivity and message passing in an end-to-end fashion. We evaluate our model an outcome prediction task on a Tuberculosis (TB) dataset consistently outperforming several state-of-the-art neural, graph-based and traditional fusion techniques.

**Keywords:** Multimodal Fusion · Hirschfeld-Gebelein-Reñyi (HGR) maximal correlation · Multi-Layered Graphs · Multi-Graph Neural Networks

## 1 Introduction

In the age of modern medicine, it is now possible to capture information about a patient through multiple data-rich modalities to give a holistic view of a patient's condition. In complex diseases such as cancer [18], tuberculosis [16] or autism spectrum disorder [7–9], evidence for a diagnosis or treatment outcome may be

A. K. Maier et al. (Eds.): ML4MHD 2023, LNCS 14315, pp. 141–154, 2024.
https://doi.org/10.1007/978-3-031-47679-2_11

present in multiple modalities such as clinical, genomic, molecular, pathological and radiological imaging. Reliable patient-tailored outcome prediction requires fusing information from modality data both within and across patients. This can be achieved by effectively modeling the fine-grained and multi-faceted complex interactions between modality features. In general, this is a challenging problem as it is largely unclear what information is best captured by each modality, how best to combine modalities, and how to effectively extract predictive patterns from data [14].

## 1.1  Related Works

Existing attempts to fuse modalities for outcome prediction can be divided into at least three approaches, namely, feature vector-based, statistical or graph-based approaches. The vector-based approaches perform early, intermediate, or late fusion [1,18] with the late fusion approach combining the results of prediction rather than fusing the modality features. Due to the restrictive nature of the underlying assumptions, these are often inadequate for characterizing the broader range of relationships among modality features and their relevance for prediction. In statistical approaches, methods such as canonical correlation analysis [19] and its deep learning variants [25] directly model feature correlations either in the native representation or in a latent space [18]. However, these are not guaranteed to learn discriminative patterns in the unsupervised setting and can suffer from scalability issues when integrated into larger predictive models [23]. Recently, graph-based approaches have been developed which form basic [2,5,26] or multiplexed graphs [6] from latent embeddings derived from modality features using concatenation [2] or weighted averaging [26]. Task-specific fusion is then achieved through inference via message passing walks between nodes in a graph neural network. In the basic collapsed graph construction, the inter-patient and intra-patient modality correlations are not fully distinguished. Conversely, in the multiplexed formulation [6], only a restricted form of multi-relational dependence is captured between nodes through vertical connections. Since the graph is defined using latent embedding directions, the modality semantics are not preserved. Additionally, the staged training of the graph construction and inference networks do not guarantee that the constructed graphs retain discriminable interaction patterns.

## 1.2  Our Contributions

We develop a novel end-to-end fusion framework that addresses the limitations mentioned above. The Maximal Correlation Multi-Layered Graph Neural Network, i.e. MaxCorrMGNN, is a general yet interpretable framework for problems of multimodal fusion with unstructured data. Specifically, our approach marries the design principles of statistical representation learning with deep learning models for reasoning from multi-graphs.

The main contributions of this work are three-fold:

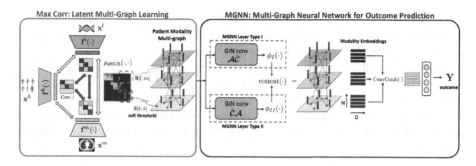

**Fig. 1.** Our Generalized Framework for Multimodal Fusion **Gray Box:** The features from different modalities are input to the MaxCorr (HGR) formulation. The nodes are the patients of the Multi-Graph, and the planes are the modalities. **Purple Box:** The Multi-Graph Neural Network maps the multi-graph representation to the targets. (Color figure online)

- First, we propose to model intra and inter-patient modality relationships explicitly through a novel patient-modality multi-layered graph as shown in Fig. 1. The edges in each layer (plane of the multi-graph) capture the *intra-modality relations* between patients, while the cross-edges between layers capture *inter-modality relations* across patients.
- Since these relationships are not known apriori for unstructured data, we propose, for the first time, to use learnable Hirschfeld-Gebelein-Reñyi (HGR) maximal correlations. We introduce learnable soft-thresholding to uncover salient connectivity patterns automatically. Effectively, this procedure allows us to express any multimodal dataset as a patient-modality multilayered graph for fusion.
- Third, we develop a multilayered graph neural network (MGNN) from first principles for task-informed reasoning from multi-layered graphs.

To demonstrate the generality of our approach, we evaluate our framework on a large Tuberculosis (TB) dataset for multi-outcome prediction. Through rigorous experimentation, we show our framework outperforms several state-of-the-art graph based and traditional fusion baselines.

## 2    MaxCorrMGNN Formulation for Multimodal Fusion

We now describe the four main aspects of our formulation, namely, (a) multilayered graph representation, (b) formalism for maximal correlation (c) task-specific inference through graph neural networks, and (d) loss function for end-to-end learning of both graph connectivity and inference.

### 2.1    Patient-Modality Multi-layered Graph

Given multimodal data about patients, we model the modality and patient information through a multi-layered graph [3] as shown in Fig. 1. *Here the nodes are grouped into multiple planes, each plane representing edge-connectivity according to an individual modality while each patient is represented by a set of corresponding nodes across the layers* (called a supra-node).

Mathematically, we represent the multi-layered graph as: $\mathcal{G}_M = (\mathcal{V}, \mathcal{E}_M)$, where $|\mathcal{V}_M| = |\mathcal{V}| \times K$ are the extended supra-nodes and $\mathcal{E}_M = \{(i, j) \in \mathcal{V}_M \times \mathcal{V}_M\}$ are the edges between supra-nodes. There are $K$ modality planes, each with adjacency matrices $\mathbf{A}_{(k)} \in \mathcal{R}^{P \times P}$. The $K \times K$ pairwise cross planar connections are given by $\mathbf{C}_{(l,m)} \in \mathcal{R}^{P \times P}$, where $P = |\mathcal{V}|$. All edge weights may take values in range $[0 - 1]$.

## 2.2  HGR Maximal Correlations for Latent Multi-graph Learning

Recall that we would like to learn task informed patient-modality multi-graph representations automatically from unstructured modality data. To this end, we develop the framework illustrated in the Gray Box in Fig. 1.

Let $\{\mathbf{x}_n^k \in \mathcal{R}^{D_k \times 1}\}_{k=1}^K$ be the features from to modality $k$ for patient $n$. Since features from different modalities lie in different input subspaces, we develop parallel common space projections to explore the dependence between them. The Hirschfield, Gebelin, Rènyi (HGR) [23] framework in statistics is known to generalize the notion of dependence to abstract and non-linear functional spaces. Such non-linear projections can be parameterized by deep neural networks.

Specifically, let the collection of modality-specific projection networks be given by $\{\mathbf{f}^k(\cdot) : \mathcal{R}^{D_k \times 1} \rightarrow \mathcal{R}^{D_p \times 1}\}$. The HGR maximal correlation is a symmetric measure obtained by solving the following coupled pairwise constrained optimization problem:

$$\sup_{\mathcal{C}_E, \mathcal{C}_{\mathrm{Cov}}} \rho_{\mathrm{HGR}}(\mathbf{x}^l, \mathbf{x}^m) = \sup_{\mathcal{C}_E, \mathcal{C}_{\mathrm{Cov}}} \mathbb{E}\Big[[\mathbf{f}^l(\mathbf{x}^l)]^T \mathbf{f}^m(\mathbf{x}^m)\Big] \tag{1}$$

$\forall \{l.m\}$ s.t. $l \neq m$, where $\mathcal{I}_{D_p}$ is a $D_p \times D_p$ identity matrix. The constraint sets are given by:

$$\mathcal{C}_E : \{\mathbb{E}[\mathbf{f}^l(\cdot)] = \mathbb{E}[\mathbf{f}^m(\cdot)] = \mathbf{0}\} \tag{2}$$

$$\mathcal{C}_{\mathrm{Cov}} : \{\mathbf{Cov}(\mathbf{f}^l(\mathbf{x}^l)) = \mathbf{Cov}(\mathbf{f}^m(\mathbf{x}^m)) = \mathcal{I}_{D_p}\} \tag{3}$$

Approaches such as deep CCA [25] can be thought of as a special case of this formulation which solve the whitening (empirical covariance) constraints (Eq. (3)) via explicit pairwise de-correlation.

However, for multiple modalities in large datasets, exact whitening is not scalable. To circumvent this issue, we can use the approach in [23]. This formulation proposes introduces a relaxation to the exact HGR, named soft-HGR, which consists of a trace regularizer in lieu of whitening. Equation (1) can be relaxed as an empirical minimization problem min $\mathcal{L}_{\mathrm{sHGR}}$, where the sHGR loss is:

$$\mathcal{L}_{\text{sHGR}} = -\frac{1}{N_z} \mathbb{E}\left[\mathbf{f}^l(\mathbf{x}^l)^T \mathbf{f}^m(\mathbf{x}^m)\right] + \frac{1}{2N_z} \text{Tr}\left[\mathbf{Cov}[\mathbf{f}^l(\mathbf{x}^l)]\mathbf{Cov}[\mathbf{f}^m(\mathbf{x}^m)]\right]$$

$$= -\frac{1}{N_z}\left(\sum_{l,m=1}^{K}\left[\sum_{n=1}^{N}\frac{\mathbf{f}^l(\mathbf{x}_n^l)^T \mathbf{f}^m(\mathbf{x}_n^m)}{(N-1)} - \frac{\text{Tr}\left[\mathbf{Cov}[\mathbf{f}^l(\mathbf{x}^l)]\mathbf{Cov}[\mathbf{f}^m(\mathbf{x}^m)]\right]}{2}\right]\right) \quad l \neq m \quad (4)$$

The expectation under the functional transformations $\mathbb{E}[\mathbf{f}^l(\mathbf{x}^l)] = \mathbb{E}[\mathbf{f}^m(\mathbf{x}^m)] = \mathbf{0}$ is enforced step-wise by mean subtraction during optimization. Here, $\mathbf{Cov}(\cdot)$ is the empirical covariance matrix. We parameterize $\{\mathbf{f}^k(\cdot)\}$ as a simple two layered fully connected neural network with a normalization factor as $N_z = M(M-1)$.

By design, the MaxCorr formulation allows us to utilize the correlation $\rho_{\text{sHGR}}(\mathbf{x}_i^l, \mathbf{x}_j^m)$ (computed after solving Eq. (4)) to model dependence between patients $i$ and $j$ according to the $l$ and $m$ modality features in a general setting. The absolute value of this correlation measure define the edge weights between nodes in the patient-modality multi-graph. As opposed to existing.

***Learnable Adaptive Sparsity:*** Additionally, we would like to have our learning framework automatically discover and retain salient edges that are relevant for prediction. To encourage sparsity in the edges, we utilize a learnable soft-thresholding formulation. We first define a symmetric block sparsity matrix $\mathbf{S}$. Since edge weights in the multi-graph are in the range $[0-1]$, we normalize it through the sigmoid function as $\tilde{\mathbf{S}} = \tilde{\mathbf{S}}^T = \text{Sigmoid}(\mathbf{S}) \in \mathcal{R}^{K \times K}$. The entries of the soft-thresholding matrix $\tilde{\mathbf{S}}[l,m]$ define learnable thresholds for the cross modal connections when $l \neq m$ and in-plane connections when $l = m$. Finally, the cross modal edges and in-plane edges of the multi-graph are given by

$$\mathbf{C}_{(l,m)}[i,j] = \text{ReLU}(\tilde{\rho}_{\text{sHGR}}(\mathbf{x}_i^l, \mathbf{x}_j^m) - \tilde{\mathbf{S}}[l,m]) \tag{5}$$

$$\mathbf{A}_k[i,j] = \text{ReLU}(\tilde{\rho}_{\text{sHGR}}(\mathbf{x}_i^k, \mathbf{x}_j^k) - \tilde{\mathbf{S}}[k,k]) \tag{6}$$

with $\tilde{\rho}_{\text{sHGR}} = |\rho_{\text{sHGR}}|$ respectively. The adjacency matrices $\mathbf{A}_{(k)}$ model the dependence within the features of modality $k$, while the cross planar matrices $\{\mathbf{C}_{(l,m)}\}$ capture interactions across modalities. Overall, $\mathbf{S}$ acts as a regularizer that suppresses noisy weak dependencies. These regularization parameters are automatically inferred during training along with the MaxCorr projection parameters $\{\mathbf{f}^k(\cdot)\}$. This effectively adds just $K(K+1)$ learnable parameters to the MaxCorrMGNN.

## 2.3 Multi-graph Neural Network

As a standalone optimization, the MaxCorr block is not guaranteed to learn discriminative projections of modality features. A natural next step is to couple the multi-graph representation learning with the classification task. Graph Neural Networks have recently become popular tools for reasoning from graphs and graph-signals. Given the patient-modality multi-graph, we design an extension of traditional graph neural networks to multi-graphs for inference tasks.

Conventional GNNs filter information based on the graph topology (i.e. the adjacency matrix) to map the node features to the targets based on graph traversals. Conceptually, cascading $l$ GNN layers is analogous to filtered information pooling at each node from its $l$-hop neighbors [13] inferred from the powers of the graph adjacency matrix. These neighborhoods can be reached by seeding walks on the graph starting at the desired node. Inspired by this design, we craft a multi-graph neural network (Purple Box in Fig. 1) for outcome prediction. Our MGNN generalizes structured message passing to the multi-graph in a manner similar to those done for multiplexed graphs [6]. Notably, our formulation is more general, as it avoids using strictly vertical interaction constraints between patients across modalities.

We first construct two supra-adjacency matrices to perform walks on the multi-graph $\mathcal{G}_M$ for fusion. The first is the *intra-modality adjacency matrix* $\mathcal{A} \in \mathcal{R}^{PK \times PK}$. The second is the *inter-modality connectivity matrix* $\mathcal{C} \in \mathcal{R}^{PK \times PK}$, each defined block-wise. Mathematically, we express this as:

$$\mathcal{A} = \bigoplus_k \mathbf{A}_{(k)} \tag{7}$$

$$\hat{\mathcal{C}} : \hat{\mathcal{C}}[lP : (l+1)P, mP : (m+1)P] = \mathbf{C}_{(l,m)} \, \mathbb{1}(l \neq m) + \mathcal{I}_P \, \mathbb{1}(l = m) \tag{8}$$

where $\bigoplus$ is the direct sum operation and $\mathbb{1}$ denotes the indicator function. By design, $\mathcal{A}$ is block-diagonal and allows for within-planar (intra-modality) transitions between nodes. The off-diagonal blocks of $\hat{\mathcal{C}}$, i.e. $\mathbf{C}_{(l,m)}$, capture transitions between nodes as per cross-planar (inter-modality) relationships.

***MGNN Message Passing Walks:*** Walks on $\mathcal{G}_M$ combine within and across planar steps to reach a patient supra-node $s_j$ from another supra-node $s_i$ $(s_i, s_j \in \mathcal{V}_M)$. We characterize the multi-hop neighborhoods and transitions using factorized operations involving $\mathcal{A}$ and $\hat{\mathcal{C}}$. We can perform a multi-graph walk via two types of distinct steps, i.e., (1) an isolated intra-planar transition or (2) a transition involving an inter-planar step either before or after a within-planar step. These steps can be exhaustively recreated via two factorizations: (I) *after* one intra-planar step, the walk *may* continue in the same modal plane or hop to a different one via $\mathcal{A}\hat{\mathcal{C}}$ and (II) the walk *may* continue in the current modal plane or hop to a different plane *before* the intra-planar step via $\hat{\mathcal{C}}\mathcal{A}$.

The Multi-Graph Neural Network (MGNN) uses these walk operations to automatically mine predictive patterns from the multi-graph given the targets (task-supervision) and the GNN parameters. For supra-node $s_i$, $\mathbf{h}_{s_i}^{(d)} \in \mathcal{R}^{D^d \times 1}$ is the feature (supra)-embedding at MGNN depth $d$. The forward pass operations of the MGNN are as follows:

$$\mathbf{h}_{s_i,I}^{(d+1)} = \phi_I^{(d)}\left((1+\epsilon)\mathbf{h}_{s_i}^{(d)} + \text{wmean}\left[\mathbf{h}_{s_j}^{(d)}, \mathcal{A}\hat{\mathcal{C}}[s_i, s_j] \; ; \; s_j \in \mathcal{N}_{\mathcal{A}\hat{\mathcal{C}}}(s_i)\right]\right) \tag{9}$$

$$\mathbf{h}_{s_i,II}^{(d+1)} = \phi_{II}^{(d)}\left((1+\epsilon)\mathbf{h}_{s_i}^{(d)} + \text{wmean}\left[\mathbf{h}_{s_j}^{(d)}, \hat{\mathcal{C}}\mathcal{A}[s_i, s_j] \; ; \; s_j \in \mathcal{N}_{\hat{\mathcal{C}}\mathcal{A}}(s_i)\right]\right) \tag{10}$$

$$\mathbf{h}_{s_i}^{(d+1)} = \text{concat}(\mathbf{h}_{s_i,I}^{(d+1)}, \mathbf{h}_{s_i,II}^{(d+1)}) \tag{11}$$

$$\mathbf{g}_o(\{\mathbf{h}_{s_i}^{(L)}\}_{s_i \leftrightarrow i}) = \hat{\mathbf{Y}}_i \tag{12}$$

At the input layer, we have $\mathbf{h}_{s_i}^{(0)} = \mathbf{f}^k(\mathbf{x}_i^k)$ computed from the modality features for patient $i$ after the sHGR transformation from the corresponding modality $k$. We then concatenate the supra-embeddings as input to the next layer i.e. $\mathbf{h}_{s_i}^{(d+1)}$. Equations (9–10) denote the Graph Isomorphism Network (GIN) [24] with $\{\phi_I^{(d)}(\cdot), \phi_{II}^{(d)}(\cdot)\}$ as layerwise linear transformations. This performs message passing on the multi-graph using the neighborhood relationships and normalized edge weights from the walk matrices in the weighted mean operation wmean($\cdot$).

From the interpretability standpoint, these *operations keep the semantics of the embeddings intact at both the patient and modality level throughout the MaxCorrMGNN transformations.* Finally, $\mathbf{g}_o(\cdot)$ is a graph readout network that maps to the one-hot encoded outcome $\mathbf{Y}$, which performs a convex combination of the filtered modality embeddings, followed by a linear readout.

## 2.4   End-to-End Learning Through Task Supervision

Piecing together the constituent components, i.e. the latent graph learning and MGNN inference module, we optimize the following coupled objective function:

$$\mathcal{L} = \lambda \mathcal{L}_{\text{sHGR}} + (1 - \lambda)\mathcal{L}_{\text{CE}}(\hat{\mathbf{Y}}, \mathbf{Y}) \tag{13}$$

with $\lambda \in [0, 1]$ being a tradeoff parameter and $\mathcal{L}_{CE}(\cdot)$ being the cross entropy loss. The parameters $\{\{\mathbf{f}^k(\cdot)\}, \mathbf{S}, \{\phi_I^{(d)}(\cdot), \phi_{II}^{(d)}(\cdot), \epsilon\}, \mathbf{g}_o(\cdot)\}$ of the framework are jointly learned via standard backpropagation.

***Inductive Learning for Multi-graph Neural Networks:*** The multi-graph is designed to have subjects as the nodes, which requires us to adapt training to accommodate an inductive learning setup. Specifically, we train the MaxCorrMGNN in a fully supervised fashion by extending the principles outlined in [2] for multi-layered graphs. During training, we use only the supra-node features and induced sub-graph edges (including both cross-modal and intra-planar edges) associated with the subjects in the training set for backpropagation. During validation/testing, we freeze the parameter estimates and add in the edges corresponding to the unseen patients to perform a forward pass for estimation. This procedure ensures that no double dipping occurs in the hyper-parameter estimation, nor in the evaluation step. Additionally, while not the focus of this application, this procedure allows for extending prediction and training to an online setting, where new subject/modality information may dynamically become available.

***Implementation Details:*** We implement the MaxCorr projection networks $\mathbf{f}^l(\cdot)$ as a simple three layered neural network with hidden layer width of 32 and output $D_p = 64$ and LeakyReLU activation (negative slope = 0.01). The MGNN layers are Graph Isomorphism Network (GIN) [24] with ReLU activation and linear readout (width:64) and batch normalization. $\mathbf{g}_o(\cdot)$ implements a convex combination of the modality embeddings followed by a linear layer. We use the ADAMw optimizer [15] and train on a 64GB CPU RAM, 2.3 GHz 16-Core Intel i9 machine (18–20 min training time per run). We set the hyperparameters for our model (and baselines) using grid-search to $\lambda = 0.01$, learning rate $= 0.0001$, weight decay $= 0.001$, epochs $= 50$, batch size $= 128$ after pre-training the network on the sHGR loss alone for 50 epochs. All frameworks are implemented on the Deep Graph Library (v $= 0.6.2$) in PyTorch (v $= 0.10.1$) (Fig. 2).

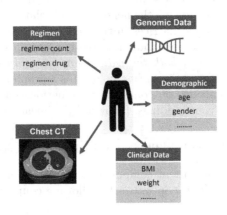

**Fig. 2.** NIH TB Dataset: Multimodal data for treatment outcome prediction.

## 3   Experiments and Results

### 3.1   Data and Preprocessing

We evaluate our model on the Tuberculosis Data Exploration Portal [10] consisting of 3051 patients with five different treatment outcomes (Died, Still on treatment, Completed, Cured, or Failure) with the class frequencies as: $0.21/0.11/0.50/0.10/0.08$ respectively and five modalities. We pre-process the data according to the procedure outlined in [6].

For each subject, we have features available from demographic, clinical, regimen and genomic recordings with chest CTs available for 1015 of them. We have a total of 4081 genomic, 29 demographic, 1726 clinical, 233 regimen features that are categorical, and 2048 imaging and 8 miscellaneous continuous features. Information that may directly be related to treatment outcomes, e.g. drug resistance type, were removed from the clinical and regimen features.

For genomic data, 81 single nucleotide polymorphisms (SNPs) from the causative organisms *Mycobacterium tuberculosis* (Mtb) known to be related to drug resistance were used. For 275 of the subjects, we also assemble the raw genome sequence from NCBI Sequence Read Archive. This provides a more fine-grained description of the biological sequences of the causative pathogen [17]. Briefly, we performed a *de novo* assembly process on each Mtb genome to yield protein and gene sequences. We utilized InterProScan [12] to further process the protein sequences and extract the functional domains, i.e. sub-sequences located within the protein's amino acid chain responsible for the enzymatic bioactivity of a protein. This provides a total of 4000 functional genomic features. Finally, for the imaging modality, the lung was segmented via multi-atlas segmentation [22] followed by a pre-trained DenseNet [11] to extract a 1024-dimensional feature vector for each axial slice intersecting the lung. The mean and maximum of each feature were then assembled to give a total of 2048 features. Missing features are imputed from the training cohort using mean imputation for all runs.

### 3.2   Evaluation Metrics

Since we have a five-class classification task, we evaluate the prediction performance of the MaxCorrMGNN and the baselines using the AU-ROC (Area Under the Receiver Operating Curve) metric. Given the prediction logits, this metric is computed both class-wise and as a weighted average. Higher per-class and overall AU-ROC indicate improved performance. For our experiments, we use 10 randomly generated train/validation/test splits with ratio 0.7/0.1/0.2 to train our model and each baseline.

Finally, statistical differences between the baselines and our method are measured according to the DeLong [4] test computed class-wise. This test is a sanity check to evaluate whether perceived differences in model performance are robust to sampling.

### 3.3   Baseline Comparisons

We perform a comprehensive evaluation of our framework for the problem of multimodal fusion. Our baseline comparisons can be grouped into three categories, namely, (1) Single Modality Predictors/ No Fusion (2) State-of-the-art Conventional including early/late/intermediate fusion and Latent-Graph Learning models from literature (3) Ablation Studies.

The ablation studies evaluate the efficacy of the three main constituents of the MaxCorrMGNN, i.e. the MaxCorr graph construction, the Multi-Graph Neural Network and the end-to-end optimization.

- **Single Modality:** For this comparison, we run predictive deep-learning models on the individual modality features without fusing them as a benchmark. We use a two layered multi-layered perception (MLP) with hidden layer widths as 400 and 20 and LeakyReLU activation (neg. slope = 0.01).

- **Early Fusion:** For early fusion, individual modality features are first concatenated and then fed through a neural network. The predictive model has the same architecture as the previous baseline.

- **Uncertainty Based Late Fusion** [21]: We combine the predictions from the individual modalities in the previous baseline using a state-of-the-art late fusion framework in [21]. This model estimates the uncertainty in the individual classifiers to improve the robustness of outcome prediction. Unlike our work, patient-modality dependence is not explicitly modeled as the modality predictions are only combined after individual modality-specific models have been trained. Hyperparameters are set according to [21].

- **Graph Based Intermediate Fusion** [6]: This is a graph based neural framework that achieved state-of-the-art performance on multimodal fusion on unstructured data. This model follows a two step procedure. For each patient, this model first converts the multimodal features into a fused binary multiplex graph (multi-graph where all blocks of $\hat{C}$ are strictly diagonal) between features. The graph connectivity is learned in an unsupervised fashion through auto-encoders. Following this, a multiplexed graph neural network is used for inference. Hyperparameters are set according to [6]. While this framework takes a graph based approach to fusion, the construction of the graph is not directly coupled with the task supervision.

- **Latent Graph Learning** [2]: This baseline was developed for fusing multimodal data for prediction. It introduces a latent patient-patient graph learning from the concatenated modality features via a graph-attention (GAT-like [20]) formulation. However, unlike our model, the feature concatenation does not distinguish between intra- and inter-modality dependence across patients i.e. it constructs a single-relational (collapsed) graph that is learned as a part of the training.

- **sHGR+ANN** [23]: This is a state-of-the-art multimodal fusion framework [23] that also utilizes the sHGR formulation to infer multi-modal data representations. However, instead of constructing a patient-modality graph, the projected features are combined via concatenation. Then, a two layered MLP (hidden size:200) maps to the outcomes, with the two objectives trained end-to-end. This baseline can be thought of as an *ablation* that evaluates the benefit of using the multi-graph neural network for fine-grained reasoning. Additionally, this and the previous framework help us evaluate the benefit of our patient-modality multi-graph representation for fusion.

- **MaxCorrMGNN w/o sHGR:** Through this comparison, we evaluate the need for using the soft HGR formulation to construct the latent multi-graph. Keeping the architectural components consistent with our model, we set $\lambda = 0$ in Eq. (13). Note that this *ablation* effectively converts the multi-graph representation learning into a modality specific self/cross attention learning, akin to graph transformers. Overall, this framework helps us evaluate the benefit of our MaxCorr formulation for latent multi-graph learning.

- **Decoupled MaxCorrMGNN:** Finally, this *ablation* is designed to examine the benefit of coupling the MaxCorr and MGNN into a coupled objective. Therefore, instead of an end-to-end training, we run the sHGR optimization first, followed by the MGNN for prediction.

### 3.4   Outcome Prediction Performance

Figure 3 illustrates the outcome prediction performance of our framework against the single modality predictors (left), state-of-the-art fusion frameworks (middle),

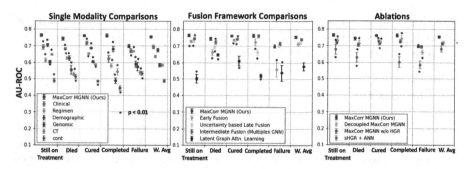

**Fig. 3.** We display the mean per-class and weighted average AU-ROC and the standard errors for TB outcome prediction against **(Left)**: Single Modality Predictors **(Middle)**: Traditional and Graph Based Fusion Frameworks **(Right)**: Ablations of the MaxCorrMGNN. * indicate comparisons against the MaxCorrMGNN according to the DeLong test that achieve statistical significance ($p < 0.01$).

and ablated versions of our model (right). Comparisons marked with $*$ achieve a statistical significance threshold of $p < 0.01$ across runs as per the DeLong test [4]. Note that our fusion framework outperforms all of the single modality predictors by a large margin. Moreover, the traditional and graph-based fusion baselines also provide improved performance against the single modality predictors. Taken together, these observations highlight the need for fusion of multiple modalities for outcome prediction in TB. This observation is consistent with findings in treatment outcome prediction literature [6,16] in TB.

The MaxCorrMGNN also provides improved performance when compared to all of the fusion baselines, with most comparisons achieving statistical significance thresholds. While the Early Fusion and Uncertainty based Late fusion [21] networks provide marked improvements over single modality predictions, but still fail to reach the performance level of our model. This is likely due to their limited ability to leverage subtle patient-specific cross-modal interactions.

On the other hand, the latent graph learning in [2] models connectivity between subjects as a part of the supervision. However, this method collapses the different types of dependence into one relation-type, which may be too restrictive for fusion applications. The intermediate fusion framework of [6] was designed to address these limitations by the use of multiplex graphs. However, the artificial separation between the graph construction and inference steps may not inherently extract discriminative multi-graph representations, which could explain the performance gap against our framework.

Finally, the three ablations, the sHGR+ANN [23], MaxCorrMGNN w/o sHGR, Decoupled MaxCorrMGNN help us systematically examine the three building blocks of our framework, i.e. MGNN and MaxCorr networks individually as well as the end-to-end training of the two blocks. We observe a notable performance drop in these baselines, which reinforces the principles we considered in carefully designing the individual components. In fact, the comparison against the Decoupled MaxCorrMGNN illustrates that coupling the two components into a single objective is key to obtaining improved representational power for predictive tasks. Taken together, our results suggest that the MaxCorrMGNN is a powerful framework for multimodal fusion of unstructured data.

# 4  Discussion

We have developed a novel multi-graph deep learning framework, i.e. the MaxCorrMGNN for generalized problems of multimodal fusion in medical data. Going one step beyond simple statistical measures, the patient-modality multi-layered graph allows us to uncover nuanced non-linear notions of dependence between modality features via the maximal correlation soft-HGR formulation. The sHGR formulation coupled with the learnable sparsity module allow us to directly translate an abstract measure of interaction across subjects and modalities in any multimodal dataset into a patient-modality multi-layered graph structure for inference. The construction of the multi-graph planes allow the node features to retain their individuality in terms of the plane (modality) and patient (node-identity) in the filtered Graph Neural Network representations. This admits more explainable intermediate representations in comparison to the baselines, i.e. provides us with the ability to explicitly reason at the granularity of both the subjects and modalities. Conversely, the graph based/traditional fusion baselines collapse this information, either in the multimodal representation or in the inference step. We believe that this added flexibility in the MaxCorrMGNN contributes to the improved generalization power in practice. Finally, all the individual components (i.e. MaxCorr, learnable soft-thresholding, MGNN message passing) are designed to be fully differentiable deep learning operations, allowing us to directly couple them end-to-end. We demonstrate in experiment that this coupling is key to generalization. As such, this model makes very mild assumptions about the nature of the multimodal data. The general principles and machinery developed in this work would likely be useful to a wide variety of applications beyond the medical realm.

*Limitations and Future Work:* In problems of multimodal fusion, especially for medical applications, data acquisition is a fairly contrived and expensive process. In many real-world modalities may often be only partially observed, missing in totality, or noisy in acquisition. Simple methods such as mean based imputation may be inadequate for fine-grained reasoning. As an aim to address this, an active line of exploration is to extend the framework to handle missing, ambiguous and erroneous data and labels within the multilayered graph representation. This may be achieved by leveraging statistical and graph theoretic tools that can be integrated directly into the message passing walks. Finally, the multi-graph and HGR construction focuses on uncovering pairwise relationships between subjects and features. A future direction would be to extend these frameworks to model complex multi-set dependencies.

## 5   Conclusion

We have introduced a novel multi-layered graph based neural framework for general inference problems in multimodal fusion. Our framework leverages the HGR MaxCorr formulation to convert unstructured multi-modal data into a patient-modality multi-graph. We design a generalized multi-graph neural network for fine-grained reasoning from this representation. Our design preserves the patient-modality semantics as a part of the architecture, making our representations more readily interpretable rather than fully black-box. The end-to-end optimization of the two components offers a viable tradeoff between flexibility, representational power, and interpretability. We demonstrate the efficacy of the MaxCorr MGNN for fusing disparate information from imaging, genomic and clinical data for outcome prediction in Tuberculosis and demonstrate consistent improvements against competing state-of-the-art baselines developed in literature. Moreover, the framework makes very few assumptions making it potentially applicable to a variety of fusion problems in other AI domains. Finally, the principles developed in this paper are general and can potentially be applied to problems well beyond multimodal fusion.

## References

1. Baltrušaitis, T., Ahuja, C., Morency, L.P.: Multimodal machine learning: a survey and taxonomy. IEEE Trans. Pattern Anal. Mach. Intell. **41**(2), 423–443 (2018)
2. Cosmo, L., Kazi, A., Ahmadi, S.-A., Navab, N., Bronstein, M.: Latent-graph learning for disease prediction. In: Martel, A.L., et al. (eds.) MICCAI 2020. LNCS, vol. 12262, pp. 643–653. Springer, Cham (2020). https://doi.org/10.1007/978-3-030-59713-9_62
3. Cozzo, E., de Arruda, G.F., Rodrigues, F.A., Moreno, Y.: Multiplex networks (2018). https://link.springer.com/10.1007/978-3-319-92255-3
4. DeLong, E.R., DeLong, D.M., Clarke-Pearson, D.L.: Comparing the areas under two or more correlated receiver operating characteristic curves: a nonparametric approach. Biometrics, 837–845 (1988)
5. Dsouza, N.S., Nebel, M.B., Crocetti, D., Robinson, J., Mostofsky, S., Venkataraman, A.: M-GCN: a multimodal graph convolutional network to integrate functional and structural connectomics data to predict multidimensional phenotypic characterizations. In: Medical Imaging with Deep Learning, pp. 119–130. PMLR (2021)
6. D'Souza, N.S., et al.: Fusing modalities by multiplexed graph neural networks for outcome prediction in tuberculosis. In: Wang, L., Dou, Q., Fletcher, P.T., Speidel, S., Li, S. (eds.) Medical Image Computing and Computer Assisted Intervention-MICCAI 2022: 25th International Conference, Singapore, 18–22 September 2022, Proceedings, Part VII, pp. 287–297. Springer, Cham (2022). https://doi.org/10.1007/978-3-031-16449-1_28
7. D'Souza, N.S., Nebel, M.B., Crocetti, D., Robinson, J., Mostofsky, S., Venkataraman, A.: A matrix autoencoder framework to align the functional and structural connectivity manifolds as guided by behavioral phenotypes. In: de Bruijne, M., et al. (eds.) MICCAI 2021. LNCS, vol. 12907, pp. 625–636. Springer, Cham (2021). https://doi.org/10.1007/978-3-030-87234-2_59

8. D'Souza, N.S., et al.: Deep sr-DDL: deep structurally regularized dynamic dictionary learning to integrate multimodal and dynamic functional connectomics data for multidimensional clinical characterizations. Neuroimage **241**, 118388 (2021)

9. D'Souza, N.S., et al.: A deep-generative hybrid model to integrate multimodal and dynamic connectivity for predicting spectrum-level deficits in autism. In: Martel, A.L., et al. (eds.) MICCAI 2020. LNCS, vol. 12267, pp. 437–447. Springer, Cham (2020). https://doi.org/10.1007/978-3-030-59728-3_43

10. Gabrielian, A., et al.: TB DEPOT (data exploration portal): a multi-domain tuberculosis data analysis resource. PLOS ONE **14**(5), e0217410 (2019). https://doi.org/10.1371/journal.pone.0217410

11. Huang, G., Liu, Z., Van Der Maaten, L., Weinberger, K.Q.: Densely connected convolutional networks. In: Proceedings of the IEEE Conference on Computer Vision and Pattern Recognition, pp. 4700–4708 (2017)

12. Jones, P., et al.: InterProScan 5: genome-scale protein function classification. Bioinf. (Oxford, England) **30**(9), 1236–1240 (2014). https://doi.org/10.1093/bioinformatics/btu031

13. Kipf, T.N., Welling, M.: Semi-supervised classification with graph convolutional networks. arXiv preprint arXiv:1609.02907 (2016)

14. Lahat, D., Adali, T., Jutten, C.: Multimodal data fusion: an overview of methods, challenges, and prospects. Proc. IEEE **103**(9), 1449–1477 (2015)

15. Loshchilov, I., Hutter, F.: Decoupled weight decay regularization. arXiv preprint arXiv:1711.05101 (2017)

16. Muñoz-Sellart, M., Cuevas, L., Tumato, M., Merid, Y., Yassin, M.: Factors associated with poor tuberculosis treatment outcome in the southern region of Ethiopia. Int. J. Tuberc. Lung Dis. **14**(8), 973–979 (2010)

17. Seabolt, E.E., et al.: OMXWare, a cloud-based platform for studying microbial life at scale, November 2019. https://arxiv.org/abs/1911.02095

18. Subramanian, V., Do, M.N., Syeda-Mahmood, T.: Multimodal fusion of imaging and genomics for lung cancer recurrence prediction. In: 2020 IEEE 17th International Symposium on Biomedical Imaging (ISBI), pp. 804–808. IEEE (2020)

19. Subramanian, V., Syeda-Mahmood, T., Do, M.N.: Multi-modality fusion using canonical correlation analysis methods: application in breast cancer survival prediction from histology and genomics. arXiv preprint arXiv:2111.13987 (2021)

20. Veličković, P., Cucurull, G., Casanova, A., Romero, A., Lio, P., Bengio, Y.: Graph attention networks. arXiv preprint arXiv:1710.10903 (2017)

21. Wang, H., Subramanian, V., Syeda-Mahmood, T.: Modeling uncertainty in multimodal fusion for lung cancer survival analysis. In: 2021 IEEE 18th International Symposium on Biomedical Imaging (ISBI), pp. 1169–1172. IEEE (2021)

22. Wang, H., Yushkevich, P.: Multi-atlas segmentation with joint label fusion and corrective learning-an open source implementation. Front. Neuroinform. **7**, 27 (2013)

23. Wang, L., et al.: An efficient approach to informative feature extraction from multimodal data. In: Proceedings of the AAAI Conference on Artificial Intelligence, vol. 33, pp. 5281–5288 (2019)

24. Xu, K., Hu, W., Leskovec, J., Jegelka, S.: How powerful are graph neural networks? arXiv preprint arXiv:1810.00826 (2018)

25. Yang, X., Liu, W., Liu, W., Tao, D.: A survey on canonical correlation analysis. IEEE Trans. Knowl. Data Eng. **33**(6), 2349–2368 (2019)

26. Zheng, S., et al.: Multi-modal graph learning for disease prediction. IEEE Trans. Med. Imaging **41**(9), 2207–2216 (2022)

# SIM-CNN: Self-supervised Individualized Multimodal Learning for Stress Prediction on Nurses Using Biosignals

Sunmin Eom⬤, Sunwoo Eom⬤, and Peter Washington[✉]⬤

University of Hawaii at Mānoa, Honolulu, HI 96822, USA
pyw@hawaii.edu
https://peterwashington.github.io

**Abstract.** Precise stress recognition from biosignals is inherently challenging due to the heterogeneous nature of stress, individual physiological differences, and scarcity of labeled data. To address these issues, we developed SIM-CNN, a self-supervised learning (SSL) method for personalized stress-recognition models using multimodal biosignals. SIM-CNN involves training a multimodal 1D convolutional neural network (CNN) that leverages SSL to utilize massive unlabeled data, optimizing individual parameters and hyperparameters for precision health. SIM-CNN is evaluated on a real-world multimodal dataset collected from nurses that consists of 1,250 h of biosignals, 83 h of which are explicitly labeled with stress levels. SIM-CNN is pre-trained on the unlabeled biosignal data with next-step time series forecasting and fine-tuned on the labeled data for stress classification. Compared to SVMs and baseline CNNs with an identical architecture but without self-supervised pre-training, SIM-CNN shows clear improvements in the average AUC and accuracy, but a further examination of the data also suggests some intrinsic limitations of patient-specific stress recognition using biosignals recorded in the wild.

**Keywords:** Self-Supervised learning · Multimodality · Precision health · Stress · Biosignals

## 1 Introduction

Stress can negatively impact health, with prolonged exposure leading to pathological conditions including cognitive, immune, and cardiovascular abnormalities [49]. The development of wearable devices that can recognize stress in real-time is a growing field of study [35] within precision health, an emerging discipline that focuses on individualized prevention strategies, diagnoses, and treatments [38].

Traditional stress-recognition methods, such as the cortisol test, require medical testing that is too burdensome for general use and is sometimes unavailable

---

S. Eom and S. Eom—Equal Contribution.

© The Author(s), under exclusive license to Springer Nature Switzerland AG 2024
A. K. Maier et al. (Eds.): ML4MHD 2023, LNCS 14315, pp. 155–171, 2024.
https://doi.org/10.1007/978-3-031-47679-2_12

[31]. General-purpose tests with physiological data do not account for variations across individuals. While machine learning (ML) is a natural solution for this task, most ML frameworks only utilize manually-annotated data that is difficult to obtain, especially in healthcare settings due to privacy and data transfer issues [17, 20, 25].

To accurately predict stress while addressing the intrinsic challenges associated with the multifaceted and subjective nature of stress data, we developed the self-supervised individualized multimodal convolutional neural network (SIM-CNN) framework. Our proposed method fused multiple biosignals at the input level to fully account for their interactions during model training [28]. In order to consider individuals' physiological differences, we built a personalized model with optimized parameters and hyperparameters for each nurse. We utilized SSL to learn baseline representations for each subject from their large pool of unlabeled data [23]. Our methodology was evaluated on a dataset that consists of the biosignal readings of nurses during the early stages of the COVID-19 pandemic.

## 2   Related Work

### 2.1   Time Series Prediction with 1D CNNs

Much research has been conducted on predicting individuals' emotional and stress states based on physiological data using ML and deep learning methodologies [8]. Among ML models for processing time series signals, the 1D CNN is proven to be high-performing due to its ability to learn local features [1]. A concrete demonstration of the efficacy and high performance of the 1D CNN is demonstrated in the work of Santamaria-Granados et al. [36], where a 1D deep CNN is applied to the AMIGOS dataset, which examines neurophysiological signals of individuals while they view emotional videos in different social settings [26].

### 2.2   Multimodal Fusion and Machine Learning

Recent work in the field has highlighted the importance and potential of integrating multiple modalities within a single model [12], especially in the biomedical domain [39]. A number of physiological datasets incorporate diverse features such as the electrocardiogram (ECG), electrodermal activity (EDA), respiratory activity (RSP), and electroencephalogram (EEG) [32]. The three primary multimodal data fusion techniques are input-level, feature-level, and decision-level fusion.

**Early Fusion.** The early or input-level fusion method extracts and combines data before learning higher-level features deeper in the network to take into account the interaction between modalities throughout the network [28]. Despite its benefits, the early fusion process can be very intricate as raw modalities are likely to display heterogeneous characteristics [22].

**Intermediate Fusion.** The intermediate fusion method, also known as feature-level fusion, provides flexibility in merging representations either at a single layer or through multiple layers during various stages of model building. Chen et al. [3] generated a new dataset (n = 52, features = ECG, EDA, RSP) and built end-to-end multimodal deep CNN structures that enable feature-level fusion. Fouladgar et al. [7] developed CN-waterfall, a deep CNN for multimodal physiological effect detection that comprises base and general modules. In the base module, features were extracted separately, and in the general module, modalities were fused, considering uncorrelated and correlated modalities. Ross et al. [34] applied intermediate fusion to EDA and ECG data for multimodal expertise classification in adaptive simulation using various ML algorithms.

**Late Fusion.** The late fusion method, which fuses data after training individual models for each modality, is usually the simplest technique. According to Roheda et al. [33], the Bayesian rule and Dempster-Shafer fusion are among the most commonly used decision-level fusion techniques. The researchers created a new decision-level fusion model for sensors that considers the task as a combination of events and takes into account the degree of correlation among features.

## 2.3   Personalized Patient-Specific Methods

Precision health formulates tailored healthcare solutions that align with individuals' distinct characteristics, such as genetic makeup and environmental factors [13]. Following the shift in trend to precision health, machine learning research endeavors, particularly those involving biosignal data, have started to implement individualized learning approaches. Kiranyaz et al. [18] built a patient-specific 1D deep CNN with ECG data from the MIT-BIH arrhythmia database, achieving high accuracy and computational efficiency. In a similar vein, Li et al. [21] utilized ECG data to first develop a generic CNN (GCNN) by aggregating data from all patients. Then, they applied fine-tuning techniques to develop patient-specific Tuned Dedicated CNN and confirmed that TDCNN achieves higher accuracy than the baseline GCNN.

## 2.4   Self-supervised Learning

Self-supervised learning (SSL) is a broad ML paradigm of learning meaningful features from unlabeled data, and the optimal SSL method depends on the specific data type and research objective. SSL has emerged as a promising approach in various domains, such as computer vision [42] and natural language processing [47]. Its utilization in neural network pre-training is gaining popularity as it increases model performance using previously ignored unlabeled data. The framework has been actively applied to biosignal data, especially on mental state classifications [2,37]. Montero Quispe et al. [27] reviewed the application of SSL in emotion recognition models and developed both self-supervised and regular supervised CNN models for the task. In broad terms, SSL can be categorized into contrastive, generative, and adversarial learning, among other methods [23].

**Contrastive Learning.** Contrastive learning is an SSL method with an encoder trained to learn by contrasting similar and dissimilar data. Deldari et al. [6] introduced COCOA (Cross mOdality COntrastive leArning), which learns by reducing the similarity among unrelated features. They tested COCOA on five datasets (UCIHAR, SLEEPEDF, Opportunity, PAMAP2, WESAD) and demonstrated its superiority over baseline fine-tuned encoders. Kiyasseh et al. [19] developed CLOCS (Contrastive Learning of Cardiac Signals), a self-supervised pre-training technique that encourages the similarity of representations across space, time, and patients and produces individualized representations.

**Generative Learning.** Generative models reconstruct the input received in an encoder using a decoder, and they include auto-regressive models, auto-encoding models, and hybrid generative models. Chen et al. [4] built MAEEG (Masked Auto-encoder for EEG Representation Learning), a specific generative model trained to reconstruct the hidden EEG attributes. The researchers used MAEEG to pre-train the sleep EEG dataset, increasing the accuracy of the sleep stage classification model by 5%.

**Adversarial Learning.** Adversarial or generative-contrastive learning models are trained using an approach where the encoder and decoder collaborate to create adversarial data, while a discriminator distinguishes between adversarial samples and real data. Adversarial learning has found significant applications in biosignal data augmentation. For instance, Haradal et al. [10] proposed a generative adversarial network with each neural network performing similarly to recurrent neural networks (RNN) and long short-term memory (LSTM). They employed their proposed method to augment ECG and EEG data, improving biosignal classification performance.

## 3 Methods

### 3.1 Dataset Description

We trained SIM-CNN using the Nature Scientific Data dataset release entitled "A multimodal sensor dataset for continuous stress detection of nurses in a hospital" [11]. The data collection occurred in three phases in 2020 during the beginning of the COVID-19 pandemic. Nurses in their regular shifts were each given an Empatica E4 wristband, a wearable device that monitors six biometric signals, namely electrodermal activity, heart rate, skin temperature, interbeat interval, blood volume pulse, and accelerometer data. The E4 wristband transmitted the collected data to the nurse's smartphone, and the smartphone forwarded it to the analytics server. Stress detection was performed in near real-time to identify potential intervals of stress through a Random Forest (RF) model that was trained, tested, and validated on the AffectiveRoad dataset [9].

Surveys were administered for each nurse to label no-stress, medium-stress, or high-stress for each interval where the RF model detected stress. Even though the system was able to detect stress in real-time, the app collected survey responses at the end of each shift for every nurse to minimize interference. The nurses were requested to report any undetected stress intervals via their wristbands or survey responses, but none used this option. Therefore, the supposedly no-stress intervals could not be validated, leading to a substantial amount of unlabeled data. 15 nurses completed the study, and around 1,250 h of data was collected, with 171 h identified as stressful by the RF model and 83 of those hours labeled with stress levels by the nurses. To ensure anonymity and maintain the separation of individual nurse data and survey responses, a distinct identifier was assigned to each nurse.

## 3.2   Data Preprocessing

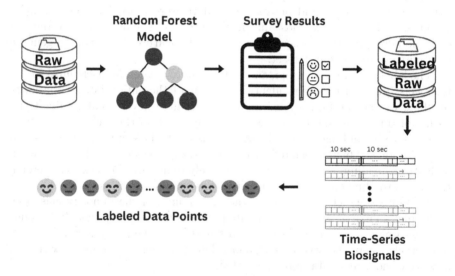

**Fig. 1.** Labeled dataset creation and data preprocessing steps performed for each nurse. The unlabeled dataset follows a similar pipeline but excludes survey results.

Figure 1 depicts the data preprocessing pipeline implemented to create the labeled dataset for each nurse. Initially, the biometric signal data of each modality for every nurse was extracted. This data was filtered to retain only the parts with matching non-null survey results, i.e., the parts that the RF model predicted as stressful and the nurses labeled with stress levels. The corresponding stress labels were extracted from the survey results and were saved along with the filtered data. We disregarded the survey results that lacked the corresponding raw data, which likely arose due to the flaws in the dataset.

There was a discrepancy between the epoch timestamps of the dataset and the start and end times of the stress-detected intervals that were in human-readable time rounded to minutes. The less-than-60-s difference caused by rounding resulted in some of the valid stress-detected intervals not being fully contained in the raw data. To eliminate this error, a minute was added to the start time and subtracted from the end time of each interval.

A 10-s window was constructed such that each sample would contain biosignal data recorded for 10 s. This data point extraction procedure was applied to both the filtered and unfiltered signals for each nurse to generate the labeled and unlabeled samples, respectively. The window size was chosen so that there was a sufficient number of data points while each data point was not excessively small. The interbeat interval was excluded from the analysis due to missing data, and the x, y, and z axes of the accelerometer were treated as three distinct modalities, resulting in seven modalities in total.

Each modality was recorded at varying frequencies, ranging from 1 Hz to 64 Hz. To ensure temporal alignment, the time series data for all modalities was interpolated or downsampled to a consistent frequency of 8 Hz. Graphs of both the original data and downsampled data were plotted to verify that no significant information was lost during this process. The downsampled data for each modality was then concatenated along the feature dimension to generate each nurse's multimodal dataset.

The labeled train, validation, and test sets were created for each nurse so that their class distributions were identical to that of the entire data of the nurse. Shuffling was not performed, as it may have resulted in data leakage due to the nature of time series data. The task originally involved three classes: no-stress, medium-stress, and high-stress. However, due to the lack of medium-stress data and the potential bias associated with differentiating between medium-stress and high-stress, medium-stress data was completely removed. The task was therefore treated as the binary classification between stress and no-stress.

To address the class imbalance, the data points in the minority class were upsampled to match the number of data points in the majority class. The minority class was the no-stress class for most nurses, as the labeled data consisted of intervals where the original RF model detected stress. Two nurses with total absence of no-stress data were eliminated.

### 3.3   Model Architecture

For each nurse, a baseline multimodal CNN model was built with the architecture presented in Fig. 2 to predict their stress level. The 1D CNN architecture was selected due to its unidirectional kernels that generally lead to performant time series models. Early fusion was implemented to concatenate all modalities over the feature dimension at the input level so the model could capture the interactions between modalities while training.

As depicted in Fig. 2, the proposed model comprises convolutional layers, max pooling layers, and dropout layers, with an average pooling layer and a dense layer added at the end for prediction. Each convolutional layer has the ReLU activation function that addresses the need for non-linearity without causing issues with gradients and backpropagation. Max pooling and average pooling layers

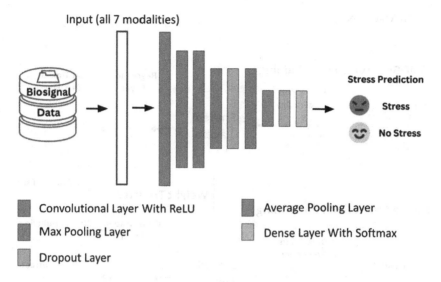

**Fig. 2.** Illustration of the baseline individualized multimodal CNN model architecture that predicts stress using biosignal data.

help reduce overfitting while downsampling the spatial dimension. Dropout layers also prevent overfitting by randomly ignoring some of the outputs of the previous layers. The final dense layer employs the softmax activation function to produce a probability distribution over the two classes: stress and no-stress.

**Hyperparameter Search and Threshold Optimization.** The initial hyperparameter search was conducted on Nurse E4, exploring variations in feature mappings (ranging from 16 to 128), kernel size (5 or 10), batch size (16, 32, or 64), learning rate (1e−4 or 1e−5), and training epochs (25, 50, or 75). The max pooling layers contained a pool size of 2, and the dropout layers had a rate of 0.3. The Adam optimizer was used to train the models. The search concluded that the optimal model architecture has a kernel size of 5 and 16 feature mappings for the first two convolutional layers and 32 feature mappings for the last convolution layer. Building upon this baseline architecture, we optimized the training hyperparameters for each nurse – namely the batch size, learning rate, and the number of training epochs – by selecting the model with the highest validation set average AUC (area under the receiver operating characteristic curve) for the last five epochs. A probability threshold is used in a binary classification model to determine the predicted class. If the probability of the stress class produced by the softmax activation function is above the threshold, our model predicts stress; otherwise, the model predicts no-stress. For each personalized model, the probability threshold that yielded the highest validation set F1 score was selected.

## 3.4   SIM-CNN

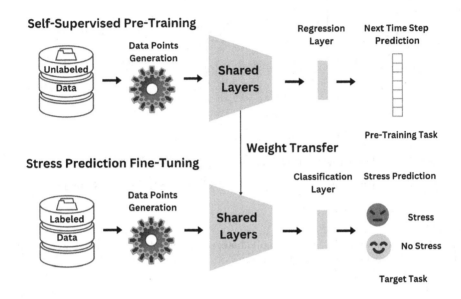

**Fig. 3.** Overview of the architecture of self-supervised individualized multimodal convolutional neural networks (SIM-CNN) pre-trained on the unlabeled data for next-step time series forecasting and fine-tuned on the labeled data for stress prediction.

**Self-supervised Pre-training.** To harness the vast amount of unlabeled data, a self-supervised pre-training task was employed to learn the various patterns in the biosignals and the interplay between different modalities. In particular, as illustrated in Fig. 3, the model was pre-trained on the unlabeled data to predict the values of the seven features for the next time step given the data for the preceding 10-s window. This pre-training task, called next-step time series forecasting, lays the foundation that would be valuable during the subsequent fine-tuning of the model for stress recognition.

**Fine-Tuning for Stress Recognition.** The model was then fine-tuned on the labeled data for the supervised stress-prediction task. A new dense layer that generates a probability distribution for classification replaced the regression layer. Compared to the baseline model, where the weights were initialized randomly, the fine-tuned model's initial weights were obtained from the self-supervised pre-training. This approach equips the model with prior knowledge about the data before fine-tuning on the labeled data, which results in improved performance over the baseline model.

**Hyperparameter Search and Threshold Optimization.** The identical architecture as the baseline CNN shown in Fig. 2 was used in SIM-CNN for each nurse to properly assess the effect of self-supervised pre-training. We searched over the pre-training hyperparameters for each individual, selecting the best-performing model and optimizing the threshold with the same methods as the baseline CNN.

# 4  Results

## 4.1  Evaluation Metrics

The metrics used to evaluate our model performance are AUC, F1 score, and accuracy. In this context, "positive" refers to the prediction of stress, and "negative" signifies otherwise. F1 score is the harmonic mean of positive predictive value (PPV) and true positive rate (TPR). PPV, or precision, represents the proportion of correctly-predicted positives among true positives and false positives. TPR, or recall, quantifies the proportion of the correctly-predicted positives among true positives and false negatives. AUC calculates the area under the TPR and false positive rate (FPR) at various thresholds, quantifying the model's ability to distinguish between the two classes at each threshold. FPR quantifies the proportion of the falsely-predicted positives among true negatives and false positives.

## 4.2  Model Performance

In order to establish performance baselines for our models, we trained Support Vector Machines (SVMs). According to the metrics presented in Table 1, there is an overall improvement in the average AUC and accuracy from SVM to the baseline CNN, as well as from the baseline CNN to SIM-CNN. The average F1 score remains consistent across the different models.

SIM-CNN overall outperforms the baseline CNN, with the average AUC improving from 58.47% to 60.96% and accuracy from 75.72% to 79.65%. Compared to SVM, SIM-CNN shows a 5.56% increase in the average AUC and a 7.95% increase in the average accuracy; the baseline CNN shows a 3.07% increase in the average AUC and 4.02% increase in the average accuracy.

The specific metrics and threshold for each nurse can be observed in Table 2, which provides a detailed view of SIM-CNN's performance. When observed on an individual basis, each SIM-CNN model demonstrates significant improvements from the baseline CNN in AUC, F1 score, and accuracy, improving up to 24.74%, 11.71%, and 15.8%, respectively. Notably, F5's SIM-CNN achieves 100% for the AUC and over 99% for the F1 score and accuracy.

SIM-CNN employs a novel method that integrates multimodality, self-supervised learning, and personalization in stress prediction on a new dataset that has not been previously used. Consequently, direct comparisons between SIM-CNN and prior research are not possible.

**Table 1.** Average of threshold and metrics on the test set across all 13 nurses.

| Model | AUC | F1 Score | Accuracy |
|---------|-------|----------|----------|
| SVM | 55.40 | 76.99 | 71.70 |
| CNN | 58.47 | 75.11 | 75.72 |
| SIM-CNN | 60.96 | 75.22 | 79.65 |

The average metrics across the nurses demonstrate SIM-CNN's superiority in stress prediction and the improvement of the baseline CNN from the SVM. However, the metrics for some nurses, namely 83, BG, 6D, 7E, and 8B, deviate from this trend. Specifically, 83, 6D, and 8B exhibit unusually low AUCs that do not improve even with the implementation of SIM-CNN. The thresholds, combined with each nurse's dataset size and class distribution shown in Table 3, help explain these results. We emphasize that all three models for 83, BG, and 8B have a threshold of 0.01, meaning that they are not successful in learning to predict the no-stress class and mostly or exclusively predict the stress class. This suggests the presence of dataset-related issues specific to these nurses.

Delving deeper into the individual datasets of the nurses whose models are underperformant, we consistently observe extreme class imbalance and limited dataset size. BG has the most imbalanced dataset, with 97.45% of the labeled data being from the stress class and containing only five samples of the no-stress class in its validation set. 8B has very small unlabeled and labeled datasets, preventing the models from learning to perform the complex stress-prediction task. Similarly, 7E's labeled dataset has the smallest size. Furthermore, 6D not only has the smallest unlabeled dataset but also has the lowest stress percent of 14.94%. This means that the RF model had a precision of 14.94% for this nurse, suggesting a significant amount of noise in the dataset. Although the specific cause of 83's low performance is not evident from Table 3, the threshold of 0.01 indicates issues within the dataset.

## 5   Discussion

We aimed to build high-performing stress-prediction models and to determine the effect of SSL on model personalization. To achieve this, we constructed a baseline individualized multimodal CNN and an identical model trained with SSL (SIM-CNN). By comparing the personalized models with each other and with the baseline SVMs, we showed that, on average, SIM-CNN outperforms the baseline CNN, and the baseline CNN outperforms SVM. For the few nurses whose metrics do not follow this pattern, we revealed that imbalanced datasets and the lack of data create a challenge for developing accurate, personalized models for these nurses.

**Table 2.** Threshold and performance metrics on the test set for each nurse.

| Nurse | Model | Threshold | AUC | F1 Score | Accuracy |
|-------|-------|-----------|-----|----------|----------|
| 3*E4 | SVM | 0.05 | 25.03 | 89.45 | 80.95 |
|  | CNN | 0.25 | 37.18 | 70.41 | 54.33 |
|  | SIM-CNN | 0.42 | 61.92 | 82.12 | 70.13 |
| 3*83 | SVM | 0.01 | 53.91 | 90.47 | 82.59 |
|  | CNN | 0.01 | 52.10 | 91.48 | 84.62 |
|  | SIM-CNN | 0.01 | 45.98 | 90.47 | 82.59 |
| 3*94 | SVM | 0.07 | 36.82 | 38.30 | 37.86 |
|  | CNN | 0.16 | 36.37 | 33.08 | 36.43 |
|  | SIM-CNN | 0.55 | 50.36 | 12.82 | 51.43 |
| 3*BG | SVM | 0.01 | 65.05 | 98.66 | 97.35 |
|  | CNN | 0.01 | 67.39 | 98.39 | 96.83 |
|  | SIM-CNN | 0.01 | 50.54 | 98.66 | 97.35 |
| 3*DF | SVM | 0.01 | 67.33 | 95.80 | 91.93 |
|  | CNN | 0.01 | 67.28 | 92.57 | 86.32 |
|  | SIM-CNN | 0.01 | 71.13 | 95.97 | 92.28 |
| 3*F5 | SVM | 0.08 | 98.10 | 96.91 | 94.05 |
|  | CNN | 0.05 | 100.00 | 99.06 | 98.21 |
|  | SIM-CNN | 0.08 | 100.00 | 99.68 | 99.40 |
| 3*6B | SVM | 0.88 | 64.27 | 63.16 | 51.23 |
|  | CNN | 0.68 | 66.30 | 75.07 | 63.52 |
|  | SIM-CNN | 0.57 | 71.22 | 70.06 | 59.02 |
| 3*6D | SVM | 0.01 | 32.21 | 24.34 | 23.12 |
|  | CNN | 0.71 | 56.83 | 11.76 | 83.87 |
|  | SIM-CNN | 0.94 | 26.97 | 6.25 | 83.87 |
| 3*7A | SVM | 0.01 | 44.20 | 97.52 | 95.16 |
|  | CNN | 0.01 | 49.46 | 95.80 | 91.94 |
|  | SIM-CNN | 0.01 | 59.97 | 97.00 | 94.19 |
| 3*7E | SVM | 0.05 | 83.53 | 69.92 | 53.75 |
|  | CNN | 0.39 | 69.26 | 74.75 | 68.75 |
|  | SIM-CNN | 0.27 | 82.28 | 80.00 | 75.00 |
| 3*8B | SVM | 0.01 | 24.05 | 80.36 | 67.16 |
|  | CNN | 0.01 | 11.72 | 80.36 | 67.16 |
|  | SIM-CNN | 0.01 | 20.52 | 80.36 | 67.16 |
| 3*15 | SVM | 0.01 | 58.92 | 97.38 | 94.90 |
|  | CNN | 0.01 | 76.67 | 97.38 | 94.90 |
|  | SIM-CNN | 0.01 | 78.71 | 97.38 | 94.90 |
| 3*5C | SVM | 0.56 | 66.80 | 58.54 | 62.01 |
|  | CNN | 0.71 | 69.53 | 56.32 | 57.54 |
|  | SIM-CNN | 0.69 | 72.83 | 67.05 | 68.16 |

**Table 3.** Summary statistics of the dataset size and class distribution of each nurse.

| Nurse | Stress Percent | No-Stress Train | No-Stress Val | Labeled | Unlabeled |
|-------|----------------|-----------------|---------------|---------|-----------|
| E4 | 80.88 | 703 | 89 | 4607 | 41805 |
| 83 | 82.68 | 340 | 43 | 2460 | 53897 |
| 94 | 29.74 | 782 | 98 | 1392 | 28943 |
| BG | 97.45 | 38 | 5 | 1884 | 27325 |
| DF | 92.81 | 162 | 21 | 2838 | 45956 |
| F5 | 94.27 | 76 | 10 | 1674 | 25032 |
| 6B | 86.17 | 268 | 34 | 2430 | 20903 |
| 6D | 14.94 | 1256 | 158 | 1848 | 8619 |
| 7A | 95.34 | 114 | 15 | 3090 | 28529 |
| 7E | 53.79 | 292 | 37 | 792 | 18236 |
| 8B | 67.35 | 344 | 44 | 1323 | 9788 |
| 15 | 95.65 | 32 | 5 | 966 | 26197 |
| 5C | 45.79 | 772 | 97 | 1782 | 35743 |

## 5.1 Limitations and Future Work

Although SIM-CNN improves the average AUC and accuracy, further investigation of the data from certain nurses whose model metrics differ from the expected pattern reveals the intrinsic limitations of precision health using in-the-wild biosignal data. Due to its inherent subjectivity and complexity, stress prediction solely based on biosignals is a difficult task for computational approaches. The real-world dataset that we used unavoidably contains biases and class imbalance, as all labeled data was collected from the time intervals that a classifier originally predicted as stressful. In addition to sampling bias, the nurses might have been biased when self-labeling the intervals since no external verification was conducted. Moreover, the nurses had to label the entire stress-detected interval with one stress level, even though it often lasted over 30 min and sometimes over 2 h, resulting in a lot of noise in the labeled data.

Combined with the individualized aspect of each model, which entails relatively smaller datasets that are more susceptible to noise, bias, and class imbalance, these complications explain why some nurses' metrics are low or distinct from the overall pattern of improvement across the three models. These issues can be mostly addressed by using larger labeled and unlabeled datasets. Collecting unlabeled biosignal data is feasible, especially in medical settings where subjects can wear devices that continuously monitor their biosignals. However, generating a substantial amount of manually-labeled data is time-consuming and costly, particularly within the healthcare domain.

To evaluate SIM-CNN's performance in the absence of these complications, it would be beneficial to train the model on a cleaner dataset with more labeled data. Such datasets can be obtained by alleviating the reliance on manual annotation, as it would reduce bias and result in more labeled data. This could also involve using data collected from subjects in professions outside of the healthcare domain since healthcare workers' data carries unique biases and noise due to irregular work shifts, the need to minimize interruptions during work hours, and other environmental factors.

There are two potential avenues to acquire such datasets. The first approach entails the presence of on-site observers who can identify stress intervals. Although this component was part of the initial design of the study that generated our dataset, it could not be realized due to the social distancing requirements imposed by the pandemic. The second approach is to gather data from individuals in professions where stress intervals can be objectively identified through external factors. For instance, one method involves the collection of pilots' biosignals in conjunction with data on flight start and end times, as well as timestamps corresponding to any warnings or unforeseen issues encountered during flights. Another method would be to collect biosignal data from service workers while concurrently recording the number of clients they attended to within each time interval. Furthermore, occupations characterized by consistent daily deadlines, such as employees involved in daily news production, present intriguing possibilities.

SIM-CNN predicts stress at a performance surpassing that of the baseline CNNs and SVMs, demonstrating its potential for effective utilization across various domains. Notably, SIM-CNN holds promise for tasks in the field of affective computing that share commonalities with stress prediction, such as emotion classification. There is also potential for transfer learning of SIM-CNN weights for stress recognition for these related tasks. Furthermore, SIM-CNN extends its application beyond mental states to the diagnosis of physical health disorders, such as epilepsy, which exhibits a strong association with physiological signals. SIM-CNN is capable of adapting the number and types of signals based on the specific task requirements, enhancing its versatility and applicability.

SIM-CNN, which implements the next-step time series forecasting, does not appear to achieve high performance without sufficient labeled data. A potential future study could involve investigating other types of SSL that could enhance model performance with limited labeled data. We could also pre-train the models using data from all subjects or explore other ways to effectively combine and utilize other subjects' data before personalizing the models. Furthermore, an updated version of SIM-CNN could be deployed into an end-to-end system designed for real-time stress recognition using a wearable device and an accompanying application.

The model personalization approach we introduce can be applied to a variety of precision health tasks beyond stress prediction. There are myriad applications in digital health where vast streams of unlabeled data are recorded with a few corresponding user-provided labels, such as continuous blood glucose monitoring systems for diabetes management [16,24,30], digital autism therapeutics [5,14, 15,29,41,44,45], and audio-based continuous monitoring of lung health [40,48]. We encourage the precision health research community to explore the application of the individualized learning framework described here to these other healthcare domains.

## 6    Conclusion

SIM-CNN is a novel personalized learning framework that integrates multiple physiological modalities while leveraging unlabeled data through self-supervised learning. This innovative approach entails constructing models with individualized parameters and hyperparameters for precision health. Such personalization of models is necessary to handle the inherent subjectivity and heterogeneity of stress data and of complex social human data more broadly [43,44,46]. SIM-CNN's performance increase in individual and average metrics underscores its potential applications in mitigating various medical complications. This performance is particularly noteworthy considering that stress encompasses multidimensional aspects beyond those depicted in biosignals, coupled with the fact that the real-world dataset that we used to evaluate SIM-CNN contains high variability. The robust performance of SIM-CNN affirms the effectiveness of using SSL to enhance stress-recognition models, thereby offering a potential solution to the intrinsic complexity of the underlying prediction task.

## References

1. Acharya, U.R., Oh, S.L., Hagiwara, Y., Tan, J.H., Adeli, H.: Deep convolutional neural network for the automated detection and diagnosis of seizure using EEG signals. Comput. Biol. Med. **100**, 270–278 (2018). https://doi.org/10.1016/j.compbiomed.2017.09.017. https://www.sciencedirect.com/science/article/pii/S0010482517303153
2. Bhatti, A., Behinaein, B., Rodenburg, D., Hungler, P., Etemad, A.: Attentive cross-modal connections for deep multimodal wearable-based emotion recognition. In: 2021 9th International Conference on Affective Computing and Intelligent Interaction Workshops and Demos (ACIIW), pp. 1–5. IEEE Computer Society, Los Alamitos, CA, USA, October 2021. https://doi.org/10.1109/ACIIW52867.2021.9666360. https://doi.ieeecomputersociety.org/10.1109/ACIIW52867.2021.9666360
3. Chen, P., et al.: An improved multi-input deep convolutional neural network for automatic emotion recognition. Front. Neurosci. **16** (2022). https://doi.org/10.3389/fnins.2022.965871. https://www.frontiersin.org/articles/10.3389/fnins.2022.965871
4. Chien, H.Y.S., Goh, H., Sandino, C.M., Cheng, J.Y.: MAEEG: masked autoencoder for EEG representation learning (2022). https://arxiv.org/abs/2211.02625
5. Daniels, J., et al.: Exploratory study examining the at-home feasibility of a wearable tool for social-affective learning in children with autism. NPJ Digit. Med. **1**(1), 32 (2018)
6. Deldari, S., Xue, H., Saeed, A., Smith, D.V., Salim, F.D.: COCOA: cross modality contrastive learning for sensor data. Proc. ACM Interact. Mob. Wearable Ubiquitous Technol. **6**(3) (2022). https://doi.org/10.1145/3550316
7. Fouladgar, N., Alirezaie, M., Främling, K.: CN-waterfall: a deep convolutional neural network for multimodal physiological affect detection. Neural Comput. Appl. **34** (2022). https://doi.org/10.1007/s00521-021-06516-3

8. Gedam, S., Paul, S.: A review on mental stress detection using wearable sensors and machine learning techniques. IEEE Access **9**, 84045–84066 (2021). https://doi.org/10.1109/ACCESS.2021.3085502

9. Haouij, N.E., Poggi, J.M., Sevestre-Ghalila, S., Ghozi, R., Jaïdane, M.: AffectiveROAD system and database to assess driver's attention. In: Proceedings of the 33rd Annual ACM Symposium on Applied Computing, SAC 2018, pp. 800–803. Association for Computing Machinery, New York, NY, USA (2018). https://doi.org/10.1145/3167132.3167395

10. Haradal, S., Hayashi, H., Uchida, S.: Biosignal data augmentation based on generative adversarial networks. In: 2018 40th Annual International Conference of the IEEE Engineering in Medicine and Biology Society (EMBC), pp. 368–371, July 2018. https://doi.org/10.1109/EMBC.2018.8512396

11. Hosseini, M., et al.: A multi-modal sensor dataset for continuous stress detection of nurses in a hospital. Sci. Data **9** (2021). https://doi.org/10.1038/s41597-022-01361-y

12. Jabeen, S., Li, X., Amin, M.S., Bourahla, O., Li, S., Jabbar, A.: A review on methods and applications in multimodal deep learning. ACM Trans. Multimedia Comput. Commun. Appl. **19**(2s) (2023). https://doi.org/10.1145/3545572

13. Johnson, K.B., et al.: Precision medicine, AI, and the future of personalized health care. Clin. Transl. Sci. **14**(1), 86–93 (2021). https://doi.org/10.1111/cts.12884. https://ascpt.onlinelibrary.wiley.com/doi/abs/10.1111/cts.12884

14. Kalantarian, H., Washington, P., Schwartz, J., Daniels, J., Haber, N., Wall, D.: A gamified mobile system for crowdsourcing video for autism research. In: 2018 IEEE International Conference on Healthcare Informatics (ICHI), pp. 350–352. IEEE (2018)

15. Kalantarian, H., Washington, P., Schwartz, J., Daniels, J., Haber, N., Wall, D.P.: Guess what? Towards understanding autism from structured video using facial affect. J. Healthcare Inf. Res. **3**, 43–66 (2019)

16. Kavakiotis, I., Tsave, O., Salifoglou, A., Maglaveras, N., Vlahavas, I., Chouvarda, I.: Machine learning and data mining methods in diabetes research. Comput. Struct. Biotechnol. J. **15**, 104–116 (2017)

17. Kim, H.H., Kim, B., Joo, S., Shin, S.Y., Cha, H.S., Park, Y.R.: Why do data users say health care data are difficult to use? A cross-sectional survey study. J. Med. Internet Res. **21**(8), e14126 (2019). https://doi.org/10.2196/14126. https://www.jmir.org/2019/8/e14126/

18. Kiranyaz, S., Ince, T., Gabbouj, M.: Real-time patient-specific ECG classification by 1-D convolutional neural networks. IEEE Trans. Biomed. Eng. **63**(3), 664–675 (2016). https://doi.org/10.1109/TBME.2015.2468589

19. Kiyasseh, D., Zhu, T., Clifton, D.: A clinical deep learning framework for continually learning from cardiac signals across diseases, time, modalities, and institutions. Nat. Commun. **12**, 4221 (2021). https://doi.org/10.1038/s41467-021-24483-0

20. Kruse, C.S., Goswamy, R., Raval, Y., Marawi, S.: Challenges and opportunities of big data in health care: a systematic review. JMIR Med. Inform. **4**(4), e38 (2016). https://doi.org/10.2196/medinform.5359. https://medinform.jmir.org/2016/4/e38/

21. Li, Y., Pang, Y., Wang, J., Li, X.: Patient-specific ECG classification by deeper CNN from generic to dedicated. Neurocomputing **314**, 336–346 (2018). https://doi.org/10.1016/j.neucom.2018.06.068. https://www.sciencedirect.com/science/article/pii/S0925231218308063

22. Liang, P.P., Zadeh, A., Morency, L.P.: Foundations and trends in multimodal machine learning: principles, challenges, and open questions (2023)

23. Liu, X., et al.: Self-supervised learning: generative or contrastive. IEEE Trans. Knowl. Data Eng. **35**(1), 857–876 (2023). https://doi.org/10.1109/TKDE.2021. 3090866

24. Makroum, M.A., Adda, M., Bouzouane, A., Ibrahim, H.: Machine learning and smart devices for diabetes management: systematic review. Sensors **22**(5), 1843 (2022)

25. Miotto, R., Wang, F., Wang, S., Jiang, X., Dudley, J.T.: Deep learning for healthcare: review, opportunities and challenges. Briefings Bioinf. **19**(6), 1236–1246 (2017). https://doi.org/10.1093/bib/bbx044

26. Miranda-Correa, J.A., Abadi, M.K., Sebe, N., Patras, I.: AMIGOS: a dataset for affect, personality and mood research on individuals and groups. IEEE Trans. Affect. Comput. **12**(2), 479–493 (2021). https://doi.org/10.1109/TAFFC.2018. 2884461

27. Montero Quispe, K.G., Utyiama, D.M.S., dos Santos, E.M., Oliveira, H.A.B.F., Souto, E.J.P.: Applying self-supervised representation learning for emotion recognition using physiological signals. Sensors **22**(23) (2022). https://doi.org/10.3390/ s22239102. https://www.mdpi.com/1424-8220/22/23/9102

28. Pawłowski, M., Wróblewska, A., Sysko-Romańczuk, S.: Effective techniques for multimodal data fusion: a comparative analysis. Sensors **23**(5) (2023). https://doi. org/10.3390/s23052381. https://www.mdpi.com/1424-8220/23/5/2381

29. Penev, Y., et al.: A mobile game platform for improving social communication in children with autism: a feasibility study. Appl. Clin. Inform. **12**(05), 1030–1040 (2021)

30. Plis, K., Bunescu, R., Marling, C., Shubrook, J., Schwartz, F.: A machine learning approach to predicting blood glucose levels for diabetes management. In: Workshops at the Twenty-Eighth AAAI Conference on Artificial Intelligence. Citeseer (2014)

31. Riley, W.J.: Health disparities: gaps in access, quality and affordability of medical care. Trans. Am. Clin. Climatol. Assoc. **123**, 167 (2012)

32. Rim, B., Sung, N.J., Min, S., Hong, M.: Deep learning in physiological signal data: a survey. Sensors **20**(4) (2020). https://doi.org/10.3390/s20040969. https://www. mdpi.com/1424-8220/20/4/969

33. Roheda, S., Krim, H., Luo, Z.Q., Wu, T.: Decision level fusion: an event driven approach. In: 2018 26th European Signal Processing Conference (EUSIPCO), pp. 2598–2602, September 2018. https://doi.org/10.23919/EUSIPCO.2018.8553412

34. Ross, K., et al.: Toward dynamically adaptive simulation: multimodal classification of user expertise using wearable devices. Sensors **19**(19) (2019). https://doi.org/ 10.3390/s19194270. https://www.mdpi.com/1424-8220/19/19/4270

35. Samson, C., Koh, A.: Stress monitoring and recent advancements in wearable biosensors. Frontiers Bioeng. Biotechnol. **8** (2020). https://doi.org/10.3389/fbioe. 2020.01037. https://www.frontiersin.org/articles/10.3389/fbioe.2020.01037

36. Santamaria-Granados, L., Munoz-Organero, M., Ramirez-González, G., Abdulhay, E., Arunkumar, N.: Using deep convolutional neural network for emotion detection on a physiological signals dataset (AMIGOS). IEEE Access **7**, 57–67 (2019). https://doi.org/10.1109/ACCESS.2018.2883213

37. Sarkar, P., Etemad, A.: Self-supervised ECG representation learning for emotion recognition. IEEE Trans. Affect. Comput. **13**(3), 1541–1554 (2022). https://doi. org/10.1109/TAFFC.2020.3014842

38. Silvera-Tawil, D., Hussain, M.S., Li, J.: Emerging technologies for precision health: an insight into sensing technologies for health and wellbeing. Smart

Health **15**, 100100 (2020). https://doi.org/10.1016/j.smhl.2019.100100. https://www.sciencedirect.com/science/article/pii/S2352648319300649

39. Stahlschmidt, S.R., Ulfenborg, B., Synnergren, J.: Multimodal deep learning for biomedical data fusion: a review. Briefings Bioinf. **23**(2) (2022). https://doi.org/10.1093/bib/bbab569

40. Vatanparvar, K., Nemati, E., Nathan, V., Rahman, M.M., Kuang, J.: CoughMatch-subject verification using cough for personal passive health monitoring. In: 2020 42nd Annual International Conference of the IEEE Engineering in Medicine & Biology Society (EMBC), pp. 5689–5695. IEEE (2020)

41. Voss, C., et al.: Effect of wearable digital intervention for improving socialization in children with autism spectrum disorder: a randomized clinical trial. JAMA Pediatr. **173**(5), 446–454 (2019)

42. Wang, X., He, K., Gupta, A.: Transitive invariance for self-supervised visual representation learning. In: 2017 IEEE International Conference on Computer Vision (ICCV), pp. 1338–1347, October 2017. https://doi.org/10.1109/ICCV.2017.149

43. Washington, P., et al.: Challenges and opportunities for machine learning classification of behavior and mental state from images. arXiv preprint arXiv:2201.11197 (2022)

44. Washington, P., et al.: Data-driven diagnostics and the potential of mobile artificial intelligence for digital therapeutic phenotyping in computational psychiatry. Biolog. Psychiatry Cogn. Neurosci. Neuroimaging **5**(8), 759–769 (2020)

45. Washington, P., et al.: SuperpowerGlass: a wearable aid for the at-home therapy of children with autism. Proc. ACM Interact. Mob. Wearable Ubiquit. Technol. **1**(3), 1–22 (2017)

46. Washington, P., Wall, D.P.: A review of and roadmap for data science and machine learning for the neuropsychiatric phenotype of autism. Ann. Rev. Biomed. Data Sci. **6** (2023)

47. Weld, D.S., Hoffmann, R., Wu, F.: Using Wikipedia to bootstrap open information extraction. SIGMOD Rec. **37**(4), 62–68 (2009). https://doi.org/10.1145/1519103.1519113

48. Xu, X., et al.: Listen2Cough: leveraging end-to-end deep learning cough detection model to enhance lung health assessment using passively sensed audio. Proc. ACM Interact. Mob. Wearable Ubiquitous Technol. **5**(1), 1–22 (2021)

49. Yaribeygi, H., Panahi, Y., Sahraei, H., Johnston, T.P., Sahebkar, A.: The impact of stress on body function: a review. EXCLI J. **16**, 1057–1072 (2017). https://doi.org/10.17179/excli2017-480. https://www.excli.de/index.php/excli/article/view/258

# InterSynth: A Semi-Synthetic Framework for Benchmarking Prescriptive Inference from Observational Data

Dominic Giles[1(✉)], Robert Gray[1], Chris Foulon[1], Guilherme Pombo[1], Tianbo Xu[1], James K. Ruffle[1], H. Rolf Jäger[2], Jorge Cardoso[2], Sebastien Ourselin[2], Geraint Rees[1], Ashwani Jha[1], and Parashkev Nachev[1(✉)]

[1] UCL Queen Square Institute of Neurology, University College London, London, UK
{dominic.giles.15,p.nachev}@ucl.ac.uk
[2] School of Biomedical Engineering and Imaging Sciences, King's College London, London, UK

**Abstract.** Treatments are prescribed to individuals in pursuit of contemporaneously unobserved outcomes, based on evidence derived from populations with historically observed treatments and outcomes. Since neither treatments nor outcomes are typically replicable in the same individual, alternatives remain counterfactual in both settings. Prescriptive fidelity therefore cannot be evaluated empirically at the individual-level, forcing reliance on lossy, group-level estimates, such as average treatment effects, that presume an implausibly low ceiling on individuation. The lack of empirical ground truths critically impedes the development of individualised prescriptive models, on which realising personalised care inevitably depends. Here we present InterSynth, a general platform for modelling biologically-plausible, empirically-informed, semi-synthetic ground truths, for the evaluation of prescriptive models operating at the individual level. InterSynth permits comprehensive simulation of heterogeneous treatment effect sizes and variability, and observed and unobserved confounding treatment allocation biases, with explicit modelling of decoupled response failure and spontaneous recovery. Operable with high-dimensional data such as high-resolution brain lesion maps, InterSynth offers a principled means of quantifying the fidelity of prescriptive models across a wide range of plausible real-world conditions. We demonstrate end-to-end use of the platform with an example employing real neuroimaging data from patients with ischaemic stroke, volume image-based succinct lesion representations, and semi-synthetic ground truths informed by functional, transcriptomic and receptomic data. We make our platform freely available to the scientific community.

**Keywords:** Prescriptive inference · Heterogeneous treatment effects

## 1 Introduction

Outside the niche area of public health, clinical interventions are chosen to maximise the probability of a successful outcome (e.g. survival, recovery, symp-

© The Author(s), under exclusive license to Springer Nature Switzerland AG 2024
A. K. Maier et al. (Eds.): ML4MHD 2023, LNCS 14315, pp. 172–188, 2024.
https://doi.org/10.1007/978-3-031-47679-2_13

tomatic relief, etc.) in the specific patient being treated. *Prescription* is therefore a task executed at the individual level, not the population, even if it relies on evidence drawn from populations [5].

Group-level estimates of interventional efficacy, typically average treatment effects (ATEs), are obtainable by randomised controlled trials (RCTs). RCTs currently define the accepted 'gold standard' in evidence-based medicine for determining whether a treatment does more good than harm [44]. For individualised treatment effect (ITE) inference, there is no such established standard. ATEs inferred from RCTs can be reasonably applied to the individual only under the assumption that the average of the studied cohort is the best available guide [34]: arguably an insult to the diversity and heterogeneity of real-world human populations. Though trial stratification and subgroup analyses can improve the individual-level specificity of such estimates, unwarranted group-average assumptions remain [13, 25].

The history of RCTs predates modern information processing capacity [33], on which methods for ITE inference with high-dimensional data depend [26, 40]. ATEs remain potentially useful where population homogeneity is artificially enforced, or where the scale of the intervention (e.g. in policy) compels a broad focus [4]. But their status as the gold standard for determining individual treatment selection decisions is increasingly hard to defend [44].

The fundamental limitation of RCTs arises from the combination of simple, inflexible statistical methods with the inadequately descriptive, low-dimensional data they necessitate. This is a defect that enhancements of the standard RCT framework could conceivably ameliorate, for example through the use of posthoc analyses for identifying treatment effect-enhanced subgroups [15], or logistic regression for inferring ITEs from RCT data [37]. Indeed, there is no theoretical reason—from a modelling perspective—not to apply ITE methods to RCT data of the size and breadth the task requires. But RCTs introduce an array of practical and ethical constraints not easily overcome. Their notoriously high cost inevitably restricts the number of studies from which prescriptive intelligence is derived [47]. Frieden [17] highlights further constraints on feasibility, such as time limitations (e.g. a rapidly evolving pandemic), or challenging recruitment (e.g. rare diseases). Moreover, the strict enrolment criteria needed to satisfy the assumption of homogeneity, such as exclusion of patients with co-morbidities or outside a specified age range, limits generalisability. Where many patients in need of treatment fall outside the inclusion criteria—a common enough eventuality—unwarranted extrapolation is the practical result even if it might not be the intention [42]. Violations of these assumptions may not only reduce individual-level fidelity but also amplify systemic patterns of healthcare inequality [9]. In certain settings, e.g. hyperacute emergency care, the complex administrative apparatus of RCTs often renders them impracticable. If RCTs remain the *sole* source of definitive treatment guidance, many treatment hypotheses will remain in the "dark matter" of evidence-based medicine, with their potential impact unrealised [17]. There is therefore a need for prescriptive inference outside the RCT paradigm, founded on routinely collected observational data, within a less rigid system of data-driven prescriptive healthcare, where clinical management can be individually optimized.

## 1.1  Evaluating the Fidelity of Prescriptive Inference

Methods for ITE inference using heterogeneous observational data are continuously being developed, relying on well-established causal frameworks [38, 43] that rest on plausible assumptions (stated in Sect. 2.1), such as that learnt treatment effects are not confounded by features predictive of treatment assignment, the risk that randomisation explicitly controls for. Methods developed for interpreting observational data as if it were randomised [22], such as the use of propensity scores for matching or weighting [41], have been reconfigured for ITE estimation, e.g. combined with tree-based methods [3, 48]. Direct estimation of ITE, in some cases with implicit propensity estimation, has been described using non-parametric tree-based methods [31], Gaussian process methods [1], representational neural networks [11, 27, 46], and 'meta-learner' combinations of methods [28].

The rapid proliferation of candidate ITE tools plausibly capable of individualised prescriptive inference has created an urgent need for a platform for comprehensive performance evaluation across realistic ranges of observational conditions. Most studies currently rely on a common benchmark database source, the Infant Health and Development Program (IHDP), first used in this context by Hill [23]. Unlike most benchmark datasets in machine learning (e.g. MNIST [29]), there cannot be a complete empirical ground truth, for unlike the case in standard supervised learning problems, here only one *potential outcome* can be observed for each individual in the dataset. For this reason, the true ITE, or true individual 'optimal treatment', cannot be empirically realised, as the outcome that would be observed if the patient had instead received an alternative treatment remains counterfactual (and unobserved). This can been referred to as the *fundamental problem of causal inference* [24].

The IHDP dataset was originally collected in the 1980s as a RCT targeting low-birth-weight, premature infants, with an intervention of childcare and home visits from a trained provider, examining its effects on cognitive test scores [7]. While falling within a very narrow clinical niche, the publication of its data, comprising a descriptive selection of covariates, has promoted a repurposing as a benchmark evaluation of ITE under heterogeneous treatment effects [23]. Most ITE inferential tools are intended for observational settings across a wide variety of domains (i.e. outside infant health), even if they are typically evaluated on IHDP data [2, 11] with or without additional datasets [26, 46]. Hill [23] adapted the RCT data by discarding portions of the treatment group according to observed demographic criteria, not at random, so as to simulate an observational study where observable features are not equally distributed between groups. *Potential outcome* responses were simulated by sampling from Gaussian distributions, parameterised by linear and non-linear combinations of standardised covariates with randomly sampled values, offset by the treatment assignment variable [23]. Curth et al. [12] has criticized the common practice of using this data for benchmark comparisons, finding systemic local advantages for some model architectures that may not extend other empirical settings.

To satisfy the need for a comprehensive benchmarking framework with diverse domain-specific capabilities, here we present InterSynth. This Python package provides a platform for the generation of semi-synthetic, fully-quantified, complete ground truths, and the comprehensive evaluation of prescriptive models in a manner that stresses generalisation. A challenging end-to-end example of its use in the context of focal brain injury is demonstrated, with high-dimensional ischaemic stroke neuroimaging data, and a multimodal semi-synthetic set of ground truths.

## 2   Problem Setup

For consistency with prior work on inference under heterogeneous treatment effects [2,11,26], we cast the inferential framework within the Neyman–Rubin causal model [36,43].

Let $D = \{\mathbf{X}_i, W_i, Y_i\}_{i=1}^n$ be an observational dataset containing $d$-dimensional vector representations, $\mathbf{X}_i \in \mathbb{R}^d$, of $n$ individuals indexed by $i$. Each individual also has an assigned intervention, represented by the binary variable $W_i \in \{0, 1\}$. The resultant outcome is represented by the binary variable $Y_i \in \{0, 1\}$. The favourable outcome is $Y_i = 1$. Each element of $D$ is assumed to be an i.i.d. sample from some distribution $\mathbb{P}(\mathbf{X}, W, Y)$.

For each individual, only one *potential outcome* can be observed: $Y_i^{(0)}$ or $Y_i^{(1)}$, when $(W_i = 0)$ or $(W_i = 1)$, respectively. The *counterfactual outcome*, $Y_i^{(1-W_i)}$, is by definition never observed, hence it is impossible to empirically evaluate the ITE, $\tau_i = Y_i^{(1)} - Y_i^{(0)}$, from which the most suitable intervention $(W_i = w_i^*)$ for patient $i$ could be inferred.

### 2.1   Assumptions

The validity of inference drawn from an observational dataset such as $D$, depends on the assumptions of *exchangeability, positivity* and *consistency* [21]. *Exchangeability*, (also referred to as *ignorability* and *unconfoundedness*), means that no unobserved confounding effects are present: $Y^{(0)}, Y^{(1)} \perp W|\mathbf{X}$. This is an untestable assumption, though it can be modelled in semi-synthetic data, as we describe in Sect. 4.1. *Positivity*, or *overlap*, means that the probability of receiving each treatment is not deterministic or fully defined by the observed features: $0 < \mathbb{P}(W = w|\mathbf{X} = \mathbf{x}) < 1$ for all $w$, $\mathbf{x}$. *Consistency*, means that interventions are *sufficiently well-defined*, where the observed outcome is subsequent to receipt of treatment defined fully by $W_i$. If these assumptions are met, $Y_i = Y_i^{(W_i)}$ for all $i$.

### 2.2   Ground Truth Modelling

The *fundamental problem of causal inference* is that $Y_i^{(1-W_i)}$ cannot be realised, resulting in ITEs, $\tau_i$, that cannot be evaluated due to their dependence on these counterfactual outcomes. This impedes the development and deployment of systems capable of inferring $\tau_i$ for previously unseen individuals, where it can be used to recommend the treatment most suitable for maximising the probability of success ($Y_i = 1$). Related work has described ITE inference within this presented problem setup [2,11,26]; our contributions here relate primarily to a framework for modelling semi-synthetic observational datasets, $D = \{\mathbf{X}_i, W_i, Y_i\}_{i=1}^n$, suited to use in this problem setup. Our framework enables explicit simulation of diverse observational data conditions, combined with empirical data, $\mathbf{X}$, and a mechanism for dealing with the *fundamental problem of causal inference* in evaluating prescriptive inferential systems.

## 3  Multimodal Prescriptive Ground Truth Modelling Using Neuroimaging Data

We present InterSynth, a platform for modelling (1) observed clinical deficits and (2) unobserved heterogeneous treatment susceptibilities given a pair of hypothetical interventions, in the context of neuroimaging lesion data. Both deficits and susceptibilities are grounded in biologically credible, anatomically-organised patterns drawn from large-scale, multi-modal data.

### 3.1  Observed Clinical Deficit Modelling

We employ a comprehensive functional parcellation of the brain [18], derived from the NeuroQuery automated meta-analytic dataset [14], to model plausible observable clinical deficits given an anatomically-defined lesion. This parcellation subdivides the intracranial grey matter (in standard Montreal Neurological Institute (MNI) co-ordinates) into 16 distinct anatomically specified *functional networks*, using voxel-based agglomerative clustering of meta-analytic functional activation patterns associated with a curated list of 2095 plausible deficit-related functional terms. The spatial clusters are associated with corresponding functional term clusters of striking cohesiveness, defining distinctive archetypal functional themes: hearing, language, introspection, cognition, mood, memory, aversion, coordination, interoception, sleep, reward, visual recognition, visual perception, spatial reasoning, motor and somatosensory.

Clinical deficits resulting from focal brain injury can thus be modelled with binary lesion maps derived from neuroimaging data by examining the intersection between the anatomical distribution of injury and the functional networks. This is facilitated by transforming each lesion map into MNI space by non-linear registration based on the source anatomical image, enabling faithful comparison across different patients. The deficit given a lesion can be conveniently rendered binary by choosing a threshold on the magnitude of the intersection between the lesion and the corresponding network (e.g. 5% [18]).

## 3.2   Unobserved Treatment Target Modelling

Just as a behavioural deficit is plausibly related to the underlying anatomical patterns of functional activation, so differential susceptibility to treatment is plausibly related to underlying anatomical patterns of neural properties. Given that stroke, like the nervous system itself, is highly heterogeneous [8], it would be unreasonable to assume interventions to be equally effective, even in the setting of identical deficits. We therefore provide a mechanism for modelling such anatomically-determined differences in susceptibility, based upon empirical gene expression distributions, *transcriptome* [20], and neurotransmitter receptor distributions, *receptome* [19]. The availability of two different empirically-driven rationales for modelling treatment susceptibility helps overcome the weaknesses in benchmarking and evaluation described by Curth et al. [12] of using a single ground truth.

**Transcriptome.** Microarray expression data from $\sim$900 anatomically located samples, each across 6 individuals, covering over 62,000 genes, are available as part of the Allen Brain Atlas [20]. Iterating through each functional network treated as a binary anatomical mask, all specifically intersecting samples were identified. Agglomerative clustering with n_clusters set to 2 was then used to subdivide each functional network into two subnetworks defined by their transcriptomic profile, simulating plausible dependence on transcription patterns of differential susceptibility to intervention within each specific network. Three-dimensional Gaussian distributions were used to interpolate across neighbouring voxels within each functional region that did not already contain explicit transcriptomic data [18].

**Receptome.** Neurotransmitter receptor anatomical distributions, derived from positron emission tomography data aggregated into serotonin, dopamine, norepinephrine, histamine, acetylcholine, cannabinoid, opioid, glutamate and GABA, are available from Hansen et al. [19]. As in Sect. 3.2, each functional network was subdivided into pairs of subnetworks with plausible differential susceptibility to treatment, now determined by receptor distributions. The subdivision was accomplished by computing the voxel-wise Z-scores of signal intensities for each receptor class, and identifying the top two classes over each functional network. Every voxel was then assigned to one of two subdivisions of its functional network dependent on which of the two values was highest. Since the source receptor maps are dense and exhibit full coverage, no interpolation was required. Division by receptor subtype (as Sect. 3.2) is also available.

## 3.3   Prescriptive Ground Truth

All the foregoing maps—deficit, lesion, transcriptome, and receptome—are defined in a common stereotactic space. This permits the creation of semi-synthetic ground truths of lesion-induced deficits and differential treatment susceptibility, the former defined by each lesion's intersection with each functional network, the latter by its intersection with each subnetwork. Concretely, let $i$ represent the index of the individual whose neuroimaging data is available in M space, and as a vector embedding denoted $\mathbf{X}_i$ (see Sect. 5). By intersecting each lesion with the functional networks, a set of observable simulated deficit profiles can be derived, and used for enrolment into synthetic interventional trials focused on a given functional domain. Within each trial, each individual thereby labelled as 'affected' can be allocated to receive one of two treatments: $(W_i = 0)$ or $(W_i = 1)$. Unobserved susceptibility to treatment can then be synthetically defined by each lesion's intersection with the corresponding pair of subnetworks, either transcriptomic or receptomic across different simulations. Note susceptibility is never conveyed to any test prescriptive model, and is here used only to set up the ground truth: it is the task of the prescriptive model implicitly to learn the associations that lead to the heterogeneous treatment effects in order to infer which treatment an unseen patient is more likely to respond to.

A critical component of any evaluative framework here is the ability to manipulate bias in the treatment assignment process, over which in the observational setting we definitionally have no control. InterSynth provides a comprehensive mechanism for this, described below, along with manipulating observational noise in modelling of non-response and spontaneous recovery described in Sect. 4.

## 4    Defining Observational Data Conditions

With a complete prescriptive ground truth semi-synthetically created, randomised and observational interventional modelling can now be performed. For each trial that individual $i$ is 'enrolled' in, the 'true' susceptibility to treatment, $w_i^*$, is available for quantifying the fidelity of inferential models. Assuming a dataset where individuals have been 'enrolled' on specific clinical criteria—e.g. presentation with a functional deficit of a specific kind—the following sections will explain the modelling process of assignment to intervention and simulation of treatment response.

### 4.1    Modelling Assignment Bias

Let $b$ represent the degree of treatment assignment bias, specified as an InterSynth hyperparameter. This is the extent to which assignment to treatment can be predicted from observed covariates, and corresponding violation of the assumption of *positivity*, or *overlap* (Sect. 2.1).

**Observed Assignment Bias.** In the context of focal brain lesions, a plausible biasing process is one determined by the morphological parameters of the lesion such as its volume and crude spatial location. Here we choose the distance between the 3D spatial co-ordinates of the centroid of each lesion and the centroid of each corresponding treatment-sensitive subnetwork. The shorter the distance, the more likely it is that a given lesion will be susceptible: biasing assignment as a function of this distance thus allows us to manipulate the influence of a plausible crude prior on the optimal treatment choice. We assume that treatment assignment, $W$, given a modelling parameter for assignment bias, $b$, is a Bernoulli random variable.

If treatment assignment bias is modelled as absent, $b_{obs} = 0$:

$$\mathbb{P}_w(W_i = w|b = b_{obs}) = 0.5, \tag{1}$$

for all $w \in \{0, 1\}$ and all $i$, as in a well-executed RCT.

If $0 < b_{obs} \leq 0.5$:

$$\text{axis} = \text{argmax}([|x_0 - x_1|, |y_0 - y_1|, |z_0 - z_1|]) \tag{2}$$

where $(x_w, y_w, z_w)$ refers to the $(x, y, z)$-coordinates of the centroid of treatment susceptibility subnetwork for $W = w$.

Individuals are then ordered (and re-indexed) according to where the centroid of the injury lies in the above-defined spatial 'axis'. They were then assigned probabilities of allocation to a specific treatment using the 'linspace' function, which evenly divides a range of values into a specified number of points.

Let $\rho_i$ denote the probability of subject $i$ being assigned to the treatment. The probabilities of allocation were systematically assigned as follows:

$$\rho_i = \text{linspace}(0.5 - b_{obs}, 0.5 + b_{obs}, N_{train})[i], \tag{3}$$

$$\mathbb{P}(W_i = w_{max}|b = b_{obs}) = \rho_i \tag{4}$$

across all $N_{train}$ images in the training set, where $w_{max}$ identifies the treatment targeting the functional subnetwork anatomically closest, on the defined axis, to the centroids of the lesions indexed last in ascending order. The assignment is then subject to stochastic Monte Carlo methods, from each probability distribution.

If $b_{obs} > 0.5$, a proportion of the lesions at the extremes of the ordered list (according to the 'axis' defined in (2)) are assigned to treatment deterministically. The degree of bias between 0.5 and 1, is rescaled, $(2b_{obs} - 1)$, to be used to define the proportion of each half of the ordered list, from the extremes towards the centre, where treatment allocation would now be fixed. Here, as above, lesions are assigned to the treatment selective for lesions affecting the network anatomically closest. The remainder, more proximal to the median, continue to be allocated according to the rationale presented above for $0 < b_{obs} \leq 0.5$, except now with

$$\rho_i = \text{linspace}(0, 1, N_{mid})[i] \tag{5}$$

across the $N_{mid}$ images in the ordered training set that are flanked by the deterministically allocated extremes of the ordered list. Treatment assignment for these central probabilities then proceeds to follow allocation as described in (4).

In these circumstances ($b_{obs} > 0.5$), the 'fixed' assignments to treatment violate the assumption of *positivity* or *overlap*; this is not a limitation. In practice, assumptions are seldom testable, hence we explicitly model violations to examine the fidelity of prescriptive models under the full range of compliance with underlying assumptions.

**Unobserved Assignment Bias.** Another assumption, *exchangability* (or *unconfoundedness, ignorability*), is that there are no unobserved confounders present. Unlike Sect. 4.1, where confounders correlated with assignment to treatment were modelled using the observable location of focal injury, here we model assignment bias resulting from unobserved confounders, impossible to predict from the data. The ability to model this untestable assumption again highlights the comprehensiveness in this evaluatory framework of prescriptive modelling.

Here, assignment bias is modelled by an information 'leak' from each $w_i^*$ variable.

Unobserved assignment bias, $b_{un\_obs} \in [0,1]$:

$$\mathbb{P}(W_i = w_i^* | b = b_{un\_obs}) = b_{un\_obs}, \qquad (6)$$

for all $i$. This ranges from deterministic assignment to $W_i \neq w_i^*$ when $b_{un\_obs} = 0$, through random when $b_{un\_obs} = 0.5$, to deterministic assignment to $W_i = w_i^*$ when $b_{un\_obs} = 1$.

### 4.2 Modelling Interventional Effects

With individuals assigned to treatments, $(W_i = w)$, and true treatment susceptibility explicitly defined, $(w_i^*)$, the observed outcomes can now be modelled. In the absence of noise, assignment to the treatment to which an individual is susceptible $(W_i = w_i^*)$ produces the favourable outcome, $(Y_i = 1)$, and assignment to the other, the unfavourable one, $(Y_i = 0)$.

The modelling of interventional effect noise can also be conceived as testing violation of the assumption of *consistency*, where the observed outcome $Y_i$, is in some cases not equivalent to $Y_i^{(W_i)}$.

Even the best-informed assignment cannot plausibly be perfect, hence we model stochasticity in the form of treatment effects (TE) that reflect the probability that the observed outcome is favourable, given that the individual was assigned treatment to which they were truly susceptible $(W_i = w_i^*)$:

$$\text{TE} = \mathbb{P}(Y = 1 | W = w^*). \qquad (7)$$

In reality, individuals may reach a favourable outcome spontaneously, whether in receipt of the optimal treatment or not. To decouple this scenario from TE, the recovery effect, RE, is applied following TE to a random proportion across the whole training set, fixing $(Y_i = 1)$, regardless of the previous state of $Y_i$:

$$\text{RE} = \mathbb{P}(Y = 1). \qquad (8)$$

**Treatment Effects.** Transient outcomes (unconfirmed until application of RE), given by the following distribution, are denoted $y_{TE}$, for TE, $t \in [0,1]$:

$$(Y|W = w^*, \text{TE} = t) \sim \text{Bernoulli}, \tag{9}$$
$$\mathbb{P}(Y = 1|W = w^*, \text{TE} = t) = t, \tag{10}$$
$$\mathbb{P}(Y = 0|W = w^*, \text{TE} = t) = 1 - t, \tag{11}$$
$$\mathbb{P}(Y = 1|W \neq w^*, \text{TE} = t) = 0, \tag{12}$$
$$\mathbb{P}(Y = 0|W \neq w^*, \text{TE} = t) = 1. \tag{13}$$

**Recovery Effects.** Following the modelling of transient outcomes with TE ($y_{TE}$), RE are subsequently applied, $r \in [0,1]$:

$$(Y|\text{RE} = r) \sim \text{Bernoulli}, \tag{14}$$
$$\mathbb{P}(Y = 1|\text{RE} = r) = r, \tag{15}$$
$$\mathbb{P}(Y = y_{TE}|\text{RE} = r) = 1 - r. \tag{16}$$

### 4.3   Ground Truth Compilation

Hence $D = \{\mathbf{X}_i, W_i, Y_i\}_{i=1}^n$ can be simulated using the empirical distribution of $\mathbf{X}$, with vectors $\mathbf{W} = (W_0, W_1, ...W_N)$ and $\mathbf{Y} = (Y_0, Y_1, ...Y_N)$ being simulated according to the above Bernoulli distributions, depending on predefined InterSynth parameters of assignment bias (observed or unobserved), TE and RE.

## 5   Lesion Phenotype Modelling

Sections 3.1 and 3.2 are conducted in anatomical space, for the deficit- and susceptibility-generating processes operate voxel-wise across volume images of functional networks, lesions, transcriptomes and receptomes. It is natural, however, for the prescriptive models evaluated on the framework to employ succinct latent representations of lesions. Here we describe a set of methods of succinctly representing $\mathbf{X}_i$

### 5.1   Raw Lesion Data

InterSynth is prototyped on an in-house empirical dataset of ischaemic stroke lesion masks, registered non-linearly to MNI space using the $b$-value $= 0$ and $b$-value $= 1000$ images from each diffusion-weighted image, and segmented with a U-Net transformer model [18]. The anatomical distribution of ischaemic damage is here captured as a binary map—injured vs healthy—covering the entire brain at $2\,\text{mm}^3$ isotropic resolution. Lesions of any kind may be used in their place as long as they occupy the same stereotactic reference frame as the other maps.

## 5.2  Disconnectome Representations

Binary lesion masks can be enriched by computing a disconnectome: a probabilistic map of anatomical territories disconnected by a given lesion [16, 45]. Such maps capture not just the anatomical region of damage but also regions affected by consequent disconnection. They can be binarised with a threshold (e.g. 0.5) and used as an alternative lesion representation within the framework presented in Sect. 3.

## 5.3  Succinct Latent Representations

From $D = \{\mathbf{X}_i, W_i, Y_i\}_{i=1}^n$, $\mathbf{X} = (\mathbf{X}_0, \mathbf{X}_1, ...\mathbf{X}_N)$ contains feature vector representations of the patient and disease phenotype. This could, theoretically, be a vector mapping to each individual voxel from the neuroimaging, though this would be unnecessarily inefficient.

InterSynth therefore offers a plug-in of any dimensionality reduction algorithm that can be used with .fit() and .transform() methods. It has been tested with UMAP [32], and the Sci-Kit Learn [39] implementations of $t$-distributed stochastic neighbour embedding ($t$-SNE), principal component analysis (PCA) and non-negative matrix factorisation (NMF). The code can easily be adapted for other representational methods, or a tabular representation of preprocessed data can alternatively be imported.

## 5.4  Atlas-Based Representations

While $\mathbf{X}$ intended to represent descriptive vectors containing covariates that suffiently capture the heterogeneous features capable of inferring ITE from, alternative representations for comparison are also implementable.

In practice, neuroimaging of stroke patients is used for diagnosis and approximate territorial localisation, when considering acute management plans. Confirmed occlusion of proximal anterior or posterior circulations is implemented into the UK practice guidance [35]. Therefore, an atlas capable of classifying lesions into these categories was sought. Liu et al. [30] released a set of volumetric atlases in template space for arterial territories, labelled according to the vascular origin at various degrees of arterial branch specificity.

Additionally, Bonkhoff et al. [6] analysed a separate dataset of ischaemic stroke lesions, providing 21 territorial clusters of distinct stroke phenotypes.

By computing the Dice coefficient of each binary lesion or disconnectome representation with each cluster (either reflected across the midline, or laterally distinct) from Bonkhoff et al. [6], and with each of the arterial territorial clusters at the four levels of branch specificity from Liu et al. [30], one-hot encoded categorisation of the territories most closely matched to each phenotype can be used as an alternative feature representation.

Lesion volume (simply the sum of the voxels segmented as ischamic or disconnected), that can be standardised with respect to the volumes within the training set by $\mathrm{vol_{norm}} = (\mathrm{vol} - \mu)/\sigma$, can be used as a standalone feature, or augmented to other representations. Similarly, the centroid co-ordinates of the lesion/disconnected regions can be used as feature representations or for augmentation.

All of these representational methods are implemented in InterSynth, applicable to any binary image in MNI space. Alternative atlases can be used as plug-ins; prescriptive performance under each representation can then be compared. This provides a platform for comparing both representational methods and prescriptive inferential methods in a unified manner.

**Representational Visualisation.** While the downstream prescriptive performance is a good measure of the capacity to represent phenotypes from neuroimaging, suitable for ITE inference, they can also be compared directly, as continuous and categorical representations. InterSynth has the functionality to plot 2-dimensional projections of phenotypic embeddings (either directly if the embedding length, $d = 2$, or following a further 2-dimensional projection such as $t$-SNE or UMAP), with colouring of the points according to their inferred category in described atlases [6,30], or indeed the functional parcellation [18]. The radius of each point can also be represented as arbitrarily proportional to volume of affected tissue. An example of this InterSynth visualisation method is demonstrated in Fig. 1.

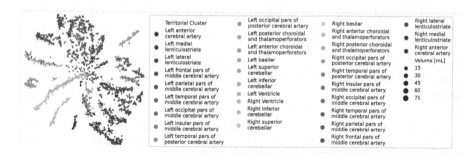

**Fig. 1.** Example visualisation of a continuous lesion phenotype representation, with each individual lesion coloured by the categorical territory (determined by Dice coefficient) from [30], and the size of each point indexing lesion volume. Here, 4119 ischaemic lesions masks are shown by the projection of their 50-component NMF embeddings to a 2-dimensional latent space by $t$-SNE.

## 6   End-to-End Framework Functionality

InterSynth is a customisable Python package capable of the above-described functionality. A brief summary of some major classes and functions will be given here: full documentation will be available with the software distribution.

generate_ground_truth() takes three arguments: lesionpath, discopath and atlases. It proceeds to iterate through either (or both) of the directories provided, loading the NIfTI images of binary lesion masks or probabilistic disconnectome distributions. For each image, the distribution of Dice scores across regions of each specified atlas (Sect. 5.4) and the proportions affected, by volume, of each functional territory from the parcellation (Sect. 3.1) is computed. This information is compiled and saved as a DataFrame.

split_ground_truth() allocates individuals to a series of K-fold crossvalidation train:test splits respected throughout the entire pipeline, including the dimensionality reduction methods for lesion phenotype representation.

embed_ground_truth() uses the above pre-saved train:test divisions to fit embedding transformation methods to the training set, and transform both the training and test sets, supplying lesion phenotypic representations of the images (Sect. 5), appending these to the pre-existing train and test DataFrames. Figures (such as Fig. 1) showing the embedding projections, coloured according to specified atlases, are also generated at this stage.

infer_deficits() assigns complete ground truth information regarding inferred functional presentation (Sect. 3.1) and treatment susceptibilities, according to either transcriptomic or receptomic data (Sect. 3.2) to each individual in the DataFrames.

prescriptive_analyses() iterates through generating synthetic treatment assignment and observed outcomes for the empirical data in the training set (Sect. 4), according to the observational data condition hyperparameters (TE, RE, assignment bias method, assignment bias severity). It is also capable of full ITE/prescriptive inferential analyses, under the problem setup outlined in Sect. 2. Here, the same train:test divisions are used, for fitting models to the simulated observational ground truth, to predict outcome given treatment. Standard inferential architectures comprising one- and two-model approaches [11] for this are implemented in InterSynth, compatible with any classifier that has SciKit-Learn-style methods: .fit() and .predict_proba(), e.g. XGBoost [10]. Any prescriptive inferential method (e.g. [26,46]) can be implemented to use the quantified semi-synthetic ground truths.

## 7    Discussion

Average treatment effects obtained from randomised controlled trials under manifestly implausible assumptions of homogeneity remain the gold standard for therapeutic inference in medicine. A shift to a more personalised approach is powerfully obstructed by the fundamentally counterfactual nature of the core inferential problem. Both model development and evaluation here requires exploration of a space of counterfactual possibility too wide to be navigated without constraint. Our proposed framework introduces suitable constraint from such empirical data as can be brought to bear on it, generating semi-synthetic ground truths that may not replicate reality but plausibly enclose it.

The approach necessarily introduces a degree of domain specificity, for the greatest empirical constraint will typically be specific to it. But the defining characteristic of the domain here—anatomically organised patterns of neural deficit and susceptibility to treatment—is widely applicable across neurology, and the complexity of the lesion-deficit and lesion-susceptibility interactions is sufficiently great rigorously to test architectures of intended utility elsewhere.

Note evaluation should not decouple representational methods from the inferential architectures; they can be complementary [27]. The InterSynth end-to-end framework evaluates combinations of representational and ITE inferential architectures for comparison, across 16 different functional deficit presentations, with 2 empirically-driven sources of heterogeneity in transcriptomic and receptomic data, and with representation by lesion mask or disconnectome. The capacity for generalisation of high-performing representational–inferential combinations, especially across the comprehensive range of observational conditions, powerfully scrutinises their capacity for individualised prescription.

The framework for modelling observational data across the ranges of TE, RE and assignment biases is generalisable to any dataset where 'true' individualised treatment effects have been plausibly modelled. Though our end-to-end framework is based on focal brain injury, the `prescriptive_analyses()` function can also operate generically.

## 7.1 Observational Vs RCT Ground Truths

Explicit modelling of assignment bias allows for RCTs to be simulated, by setting the bias hyperparameter, $b$, to 0. This means that performance of inferential architectures fitted using randomised vs observational data can be compared and quantified, revealing the conditions under which one is superior. It also offers an opportunity to explore information quantity of representation, by altering embedding length $d$ of $\mathbf{X}_i \in \mathbb{R}^d$.

## 8   Conclusion

InterSynth is a fully-featured platform for evaluating prescriptive inference models against empirically-informed semi-synthetic ground truths, with facility for manipulating observational data conditions across the range likely to obtain in real-world settings. We demonstrate its application to the challenging problem of focal brain injury in the context of high-dimensional 3D lesion data. We advocate use of our proposed framework as a rigorous method for guiding the development of prescriptive architectures and quantifying their fidelity. We suggest that closer attention to evaluative frameworks applicable to the prescriptive domain is urgently needed if we are to make progress in delivering truly individualised clinical decision-making. InterSynth, and its documentation, will be made available upon publication for research use.

**Acknowledgements.** Supported by the EPSRC (2252409), the NIHR UCLH Biomedical Research Centre (NIHR-INF-0840) and the Wellcome Trust (213038).

# References

1. Alaa, A.M., van der Schaar, M.: Bayesian nonparametric causal inference: information rates and learning algorithms. IEEE J. Select. Top. Signal Process. **12**(5), 1031–1046 (2018)
2. Alaa, A., van der Schaar, M.: Limits of estimating heterogeneous treatment effects: guidelines for practical algorithm design. In: International Conference on Machine Learning, pp. 129–138 (2018)
3. Athey, S., Tibshirani, J., Wager, S.: Generalized random forests. Ann. Statist. **47**(2), 1148–1178 (2019)
4. Beaulieu-Jones, B.K., et al.: Examining the use of real-world evidence in the regulatory process. Clin. Pharmacol. Therap. **107**(4), 843–852 (2020)
5. Bica, I., Alaa, A.M., Lambert, C., van der Schaar, M.: From real-world patient data to individualized treatment effects using machine learning: current and future methods to address underlying challenges. Clin. Pharmacol. Therap. **109**(1), 87–100 (2021)
6. Bonkhoff, A.K., et al.: Reclassifying stroke lesion anatomy. Cortex **145**, 1–12 (2021)
7. Brooks-Gunn, J., Liaw, F.R., Klebanov, P.K.: Effects of early intervention on cognitive function of low birth weight preterm infants. J. Pediatr. **120**(3), 350–359 (1992)
8. Bustamante, A., et al.: Ischemic stroke outcome: a review of the influence of post-stroke complications within the different scenarios of stroke care. Eur. J. Internal Med. **29**, 9–21 (2016)
9. Carruthers, R., et al.: Representational ethical model calibration. NPJ Digit. Med. **5**(1), 170 (2022)
10. Chen, T., Guestrin, C.: XGBoost: a scalable tree boosting system. In: Proceedings of the 22nd ACM SIGKDD International Conference on Knowledge Discovery and Data Mining, pp. 785–794 (2016)
11. Curth, A., van der Schaar, M.: Nonparametric estimation of heterogeneous treatment effects: from theory to learning algorithms. In: International Conference on Artificial Intelligence and Statistics, pp. 1810–1818. PMLR (2021)
12. Curth, A., Svensson, D., Weatherall, J., van der Schaar, M.: Really Doing Great at Estimating CATE? A Critical Look at ML Benchmarking Practices in Treatment Effect Estimation (2021)
13. Deaton, A., Cartwright, N.: Understanding and misunderstanding randomized controlled trials. Soc. Sci. Med. **210**, 2–21 (2018)
14. Dockès, J., et al.: NeuroQuery, comprehensive meta-analysis of human brain mapping. eLife **9**, e53385 (2020)
15. Foster, J.C., Taylor, J.M.G., Ruberg, S.J.: Subgroup identification from randomized clinical trial data. Statist. Med. **30**(24), 2867–2880 (2011). https://doi.org/10.1002/sim.4322
16. Foulon, C., et al.: Advanced lesion symptom mapping analyses and implementation as BCBtoolkit. GigaScience **7**(3), giy004 (2018)
17. Frieden, T.R.: Evidence for health decision making-beyond randomized, controlled trials. N. Engl. J. Med. **377**(5), 465–475 (2017)
18. Giles, D., et al.: Individualised Prescriptive Inference in Ischaemic Stroke. arXiv preprint arXiv:2301.10748 (2023). https://doi.org/10.48550/ARXIV.2301.10748
19. Hansen, J.Y., et al.: Bratislav: mapping neurotransmitter systems to the structural and functional organization of the human neocortex. Nat. Neurosci. **25**(11), 1569–1581 (2022). https://doi.org/10.1038/s41593-022-01186-3

20. Hawrylycz, M.J., et al.: An anatomically comprehensive atlas of the adult human brain transcriptome. Nature **489**(7416), 391–399 (2012). https://doi.org/10.1038/nature11405
21. Hernán, M.A., Robins, J.M.: Causal Inference: What If (2020)
22. Hernán, M.A., Robins, J.M.: Using big data to emulate a target trial when a randomized trial is not available. Am. J. Epidemiol. **183**(8), 758–764 (2016)
23. Hill, J.L.: Bayesian nonparametric modeling for causal inference. J. Comput. Graph. Statist. **20**(1), 217–240 (2011). https://doi.org/10.1198/jcgs.2010.08162
24. Holland, P.W.: Statistics and causal inference. J. Am. Statist. Assoc. **81**(396), 945–960 (1986)
25. Horwitz, R.I., Hayes-Conroy, A., Caricchio, R., Singer, B.H.: From evidence based medicine to medicine based evidence. Am. J. Med. **130**(11), 1246–1250 (2017)
26. Johansson, F., Shalit, U., Sontag, D.: Learning representations for counterfactual inference. In: International Conference on Machine Learning, pp. 3020–3029. PMLR (2016)
27. Johansson, F.D., Shalit, U., Kallus, N., Sontag, D.: Generalization bounds and representation learning for estimation of potential outcomes and causal effects. J. Mach. Learn. Res. **23**(1), 7489–7538 (2022)
28. Künzel, S.R., Sekhon, J.S., Bickel, P.J., Yu, B.: Metalearners for estimating heterogeneous treatment effects using machine learning. Proc. Natl. Acad. Sci. **116**(10), 4156–4165 (2019)
29. LeCun, Y.: The MNIST Database of Handwritten Digits (1998)
30. Liu, C.F., et al.: Digital 3d brain MRI arterial territories atlas. Scientific Data **10**(1), 1–17 (2023)
31. Lu, M., Sadiq, S., Feaster, D.J., Ishwaran, H.: Estimating individual treatment effect in observational data using random forest methods. J. Comput. Graph. Statist. **27**(1), 209–219 (2018). https://doi.org/10.1080/10618600.2017.1356325
32. McInnes, L., Healy, J., Melville, J.: UMAP: Uniform Manifold Approximation and Projection for Dimension Reduction (2018)
33. Meldrum, M.L.: A brief history of the randomized controlled trial: from oranges and lemons to the gold standard. Hematol./Oncol. Clin. N. Am. **14**(4), 745–760 (2000)
34. Mulder, R., et al.: The limitations of using randomised controlled trials as a basis for developing treatment guidelines. Evid. Based Mental Health **21**(1), 4–6 (2017)
35. National Institute for Health and Care Excellence. Stroke and Transient Ischaemic Attack in Over 16s: Diagnosis and Initial Management (2019). https://www.nice.org.uk/guidance/ng128
36. Neyman, J.S.: On the application of probability theory to agricultural experiments, essay on principles, section 9 (translated and edited by DM dabrowska and TP speed, statistical science (1990), **5**, 465–480) Statist. Sci. **10**, 1–51 (1923)
37. Nguyen, T.L., Collins, G.S., Landais, P., Le Manach, Y.: Counterfactual clinical prediction models could help to infer individualized treatment effects in randomized controlled trials-an illustration with the international stroke trial. J. Clin. Epidemiol. **125**, 47–56 (2020)
38. Pearl, J.: Causality. Cambridge University Press (2009)
39. Pedregosa, F., et al.: Scikit-learn: machine learning in python. J. Mach. Learn. Res. **12**, 2825–2830 (2011)
40. Qiu, Y., Tao, J., Zhou, X.H.: Inference of heterogeneous treatment effects using observational data with high-dimensional covariates. J. Roy. Statist. Soc. Ser. B: Statist. Methodol. **83**(5), 1016–1043 (2021)

41. Rosenbaum, P.R., Rubin, D.B.: The central role of the propensity score in observational studies for causal effects. Biometrika **70**(1), 41–55 (1983)

42. Rothwell, P.M.: External validity of randomised controlled trials: "to whom do the results of this trial apply?" The Lancet **365**(9453), 82–93 (2005)

43. Rubin, D.B.: Estimating causal effects of treatments in randomized and nonrandomized studies. J. Educ. Psychol. **66**(5), 688 (1974)

44. Sackett, D.L., Rosenberg, W.M., Gray, J.M., Haynes, R.B., Richardson, W.S.: Evidence based medicine: what it is and what it isn't. BMJ **312**(7023), 71–72 (1996)

45. Thiebaut de Schotten, M., Foulon, C., Nachev, P.: Brain disconnections link structural connectivity with function and behaviour. Nat. Commun. **11**(1), 5094 (2020). https://doi.org/10.1038/s41467-020-18920-9

46. Shalit, U., Johansson, F.D., Sontag, D.: Estimating individual treatment effect: generalization bounds and algorithms. In: International Conference on Machine Learning, pp. 3076–3085. PMLR (2017)

47. Speich, B., et al.: Systematic review on costs and resource use of randomized clinical trials shows a lack of transparent and comprehensive data. J. Clin. Epidemiol. **96**, 1–11 (2018)

48. Wager, S., Athey, S.: Estimation and inference of heterogeneous treatment effects using random forests. J. Am. Statist. Assoc. **113**(523), 1228–1242 (2018)

# Author Index

A. K. Maier et al. (Eds.): ML4MHD 2023, LNCS 14315, pp. 189–190, 2024.
https://doi.org/10.1007/978-3-031-47679-2

Printed in the United States
by Baker & Taylor Publisher Services